RECENT TRENDS IN MEDICAL EDUCATION

RECENT MACY FOUNDATION
PUBLICATIONS

Advances in American Medicine: Essays at the Bicentennial,
edited by John Z. Bowers and Elizabeth F. Purcell

A Half-Century of American Medical Education: 1920–1970, by
Vernon W. Lippard

The University Medical Center and the Metropolis, edited by
Eli Ginzberg and Alice M. Yohalem

Teaching the Basic Medical Sciences: Human Biology, edited by
John Z. Bowers and Elizabeth F. Purcell

IN PRESS

Campus Health Program, edited by Willard Dalrymple and
Elizabeth F. Purcell

A complete catalogue of books
in print will be sent upon request.

Edited by
ELIZABETH F. PURCELL

RECENT TRENDS IN MEDICAL EDUCATION

REPORT OF A MACY CONFERENCE

Josiah Macy, Jr. Foundation
One Rockefeller Plaza, New York, New York 10020

©1976 Josiah Macy, Jr. Foundation
All rights reserved
LIBRARY OF CONGRESS CATALOG NUMBER 76-40568
ISBN: 0-914362-18-6
Manufactured by Port City Press, Baltimore, Maryland
Distributed by the Independent Publishers Group
14 Vanderventer Avenue, Port Washington, New York, 11050

Contents

❦

46226

Foreword

During the 1960s a combination of factors, ranging from social and political forces to the accelerated evolution of the biological sciences, resulted in the widespread reorganization of curricula in the medical schools of the United States. A study of these developments undertaken by the Macy Foundation in 1970 led to a conference the following year, a report of which was published in 1972 entitled *The Changing Medical Curriculum.*

After a five-year interval the foundation again conducted a survey of medical schools in the United States and Canada to determine more recent trends in medical education, and a conference was convened in Aspen, Colorado, in September 1975 to consider innovations taking place in the schools and future directions of education at all levels—from premedical studies through postgraduate medical training.

This volume contains the edited presentations given at the conference, as well as summaries of the discussions. The authors, representing individual medical schools or organizations involved with medical education, deal with many of the more challenging developments now taking place in the organization and content of medical education in this country and in Canada.

John Z. Bowers, M. D.
President
Josiah Macy, Jr. Foundation

8 July 1976

vii

Recent Trends in Medical Education: Report of a Survey

MARY E. CUNNANE

In December of 1974 the Macy Foundation sent a letter to the deans of 128 medical schools in the United States and Canada asking them to describe changes since 1970 in the following four areas of medical education.

1. The admissions process: including premedical requirements; evaluation of applicants; and the significance of the Medical College Admission Test (MCAT).

2. Quality and quantity of medical school applicants; characteristics of medical students.

3. The effectiveness of the new curriculum as judged by students and faculty. Has it endured? (Personal observations will be welcome.)

4. Evaluation procedures and examinations.

We received replies from ninety-seven schools, including ten in Canada. A number answered at length, with supporting documentation; others very briefly; several responded in depth to only one or two questions. A good many replies included, as requested, personal observations about the situation at the correspondents' schools.

While the format of the inquiry did not elicit replies that lend themselves easily to tabulation, a review of the material does enable one to discern some of the major trends in medical education in 1975.

THE ADMISSIONS PROCESS

The majority of schools reported few if any changes in premedical admissions requirements. Many noted the intense competition

1

among undergraduates, who realize they have only one chance in three of being admitted to medical school. Twelve schools—Case-Western Reserve, Columbia, Cornell, Duke, Johns Hopkins, Harvard, Stanford and Yale universities, and the universities of Chicago, Pennsylvania, Pittsburgh and Washington—have formed a consortium, one of whose goals is to draw up a statement on admissions requirements, emphasizing such factors as motivation, experience, and breadth as being qualities they look for in potential students. By so doing, these schools hope to reduce the pressure on undergraduates to achieve straight As.

Sixty schools described the role of the MCAT in their admissions process. Of these, forty-two stated that the test, especially the verbal and general information sections, had declined in importance; three had waived the MCAT entirely; and one stated that although applicants were required to take the test, the schools did not use it in assessment. Fourteen reported that the science and quantitative ability sections continued or had begun to be of major importance.

Schools that consider the MCAT to be significant appear to believe it is a valid predictor of performance. With the increase in the number of highly qualified applicants, these schools contend that objective criteria are of paramount importance in the admissions process.

Many of the respondents who referred to a decline in the importance of the MCAT reported that they used it, if at all, as a weighted factor in a formula that includes the grade point average (GPA); the science GPA; applicants' personal statements; interviews; and letters of evaluation from undergraduate instructors and premedical advisors. In this context the MCAT serves, for example, as a method of evaluating an undergraduate program with which the admissions committee may not be familiar, or of immediately identifying students who will do very well or very poorly. It does not, however, reveal a great deal about the majority of students who fall between these two extremes, nor does it assist in evaluating those qualities such as compassion, motivation, and dedication, which are as vital to the education of the physician as scholastic ability.

Many of the schools look forward to the discontinuance of the MCAT, and its replacement in the spring of 1977 with what is tentatively called the Medical College Admissions Assessment Program (MCAAP). This examination will consist of five parts, including three science subsections (biology, chemistry, and physics), a mathematics section, and a reading section. In general, the MCAAP will be less factual and more problem-oriented in nature than the MCAT.

Sixty-five schools mentioned the role of the interview. Thirty-nine reported it as unchanged in significance since 1970; seventeen said it had increased in importance; and nine maintained that it had decreased or had shifted in importance because they interviewed more selectively. It is probably safe to conclude that in those schools where the role of the interview has not changed, it continues to occupy a prominent position; it is a matter of record that in 1974–75 between 90 and 100 percent of first-year students in 109 schools had been interviewed.

In those schools where the interview had increased in importance, the respondents stated that the quality of the applicants was so high, overall, that they could now be more discriminating in the evaluation of nonacademic criteria such as extracurricular activities, and, as mentioned earlier, motivation, dedication, and compassion.

Among other developments noted in the admissions process are: a trend toward computerization, including the utilization of the American Medical College Application Service (AMCAS); enlargement of admissions committees, in many cases to include students; and the admission of high school seniors to five- to seven-year programs—twelve medical schools now have such an arrangement.

QUANTITY AND QUALITY OF APPLICANTS

The most obvious phenomenon is the almost twofold rise in the number of applicants over the past five years: in 1970–71, 24,987 students filed 148,787 applications; in 1974–75 over forty-two thousand filed some three hundred and fifty thousand applications.

Accompanying this increase in numbers has been an upsurge in the academic quality of applicants, as judged by their GPAs and MCAT scores. Virtually all schools reported a steady improvement in the quality of the academic credentials of their applicants. Some questioned the validity of the GPAs, however, citing a tendency at the undergraduate level to inflate grades. On the other hand, it was pointed out that, as the rise in GPAs is paralleled by better MCAT scores, the GPA must reflect, to some extent at least, increased ability.

Overall, the replies indicate that the applicants are a more diverse group: more students have liberal arts backgrounds; a larger number are older, and more have advanced degrees.

⌐ The number of female applicants has risen markedly in the last five years. From a level of 10 percent in the 1960s, the number of women enrolled in the first year of medical school increased to 22 percent by 1973. In 1974–75 two schools reported that women constituted approximately one-third of their entering classes; one school predicted that close to 40 percent of its 1975–76 first-year class would be female.

There is some evidence that the sharp growth in the number of minority group applicants during the early 1970s may have leveled off. Several schools stated that the number of self-identified, ethnic minority applicants had actually decreased. One reason for this may be the expanded opportunities for minorities in professions where relatively high salary levels can be reached earlier than in medicine. In this connection is was noted that in some schools the term "socioeconomically disadvantaged" is replacing "ethnic minority."

Where subjective observations were offered by respondents on the quality of the applicants, the consensus seems to be that the present generation is more serious and more goal-oriented than those of the late 1960s and early 1970s. They are considered to be better students, and thus, in the opinion of some, easier to teach. They are concerned about the nation's health care needs, and many express the desire to practice primary care medicine.

THE CURRICULUM

At the Macy Conference on the Changing Medical Curriculum in 1971, Vernon W. Lippard reported on the results of a questionnaire sent to ninety-seven medical schools and six schools of basic science.

On the basis of a 100 percent response, Lippard noted that with few exceptions the traditional division between two years of pre-clinical and two years of clinical studies had been eliminated, and that there was a tendency toward early clinical experience; a 25 to 33 percent reduction in basic science instruction time; the adoption of interdepartmental instruction; an increase in elective courses; and a shortening of the curriculum to three years.

The thrust of our recent inquiry was to discover how well those innovations, which formed the "new curriculum," had stood up.

As mentioned earlier, the format of the survey was informal, as was Lippard's—no check-off list was provided to enable a precise quantitative assessment. Nevertheless, an attempt was made to tabulate, as far as possible, the responses to questions concerning the curriculum.

To begin with, approximately one-third of the schools reported "no major changes" in their curricula since 1970. These schools did, however, include those whose curricula had been revised prior to 1970; those with traditional programs that had never been revised; and new schools whose curricula had only recently been implemented.

Of the sixty-six schools reporting major changes, eight stated that the time devoted to basic science instruction had been decreased; an equal number stated that such time had been expanded. In about one-quarter of the sixty-six there was more elective time than in 1970; in ten schools there was less—principally during the first two years, when it was felt that students did not make the best use of elective opportunities.

Ten schools noted that interdepartmental courses, such as cell biology or the nervous system, had been introduced or, where they existed, expanded; eight maintained that efforts in this area had not always been successful, and that some of these courses had been dropped.

The introduction of an accelerated three-year curriculum was reported by eight schools, three of which offered an optional fourth year. In total, approximately one-third of the medical schools now have accelerated programs that enable at least some students to graduate in three to three-and-one-half years. Our inquiry indicates a trend toward a return to a four-year program, however: several schools with an optional fourth year stated that a growing number of students are choosing the longer route—and not always because of academic difficulties; two schools reported they had changed from a three- to a four-year curriculum; in two four-year schools the faculty had rejected plans for an accelerated program; and in four three-year schools there were strong sentiments among the faculty for a return to the longer curriculum.

Seven schools had established offices or departments of medical education. Several stated that one of the real benefits of the new curriculum was the introduction of modern teaching methods and instructional theory.

Among other curricular developments of the last five years, which for the most part have been judged effective, are: early introduction of clinical experience; an increase in family practice courses; and introduction of computerized self-instruction and independent study programs.

In general, those schools that remain enthusiastic about the new curriculum believe its greatest value has been in meeting the need for more personalized and flexible instruction, and for more contact between students and faculty.

Those that expressed reservations about recent innovations do not, on the whole, dispute these advantages. Rather, they mention, for example, the faculty fatigue and poor preparation that is sometimes engendered by the compression of time devoted to the basic sciences, and the difficulties encountered, not the least of which is departmental loyalty, in implementing interdisciplinary courses.

With few exceptions, schools that have introduced a revised curriculum feel it has endured, and many are enthusiastic. At the same time a discernible effort is being made to scrutinize it carefully and to make some modifications—to allow the pendulum to swing back somewhat from the outer point it has reached.

EVALUATION AND EXAMINATION

One-third of the schools reported no change in this area since 1970. A study of the balance of the replies indicates that the most pervasive innovation has been the adoption of a pass-fail system, with narrative reports given by instructors; sixteen schools had adopted such a method. As of 1974–75 only twenty-eight schools in the United States "ranked" their students. Six of the twenty-eight were, however, contemplating a return to letter or numerical grading, and six others had actually done so, citing the need for more differentiation among students, and the difficulty hospitals face in discriminating among candidates for residencies.

Comments on the present use of the examinations of the National Board of Medical Examiners (NBME), and on proposed changes in them, were decidedly mixed. (Robert Chase will expand on the current status of the NBME.)

Interest appears to remain high in other new methods, including computerized self-assessment; the development of criterion-based examinations; and the use of comprehensive tests in interdisciplinary courses.

A report of the results of this survey would not be complete without addressing some of the issues raised that do not fall strictly within the parameters provided: Whether and to what extent does a curriculum affect career choice and geographic distribution? What effect does the expanding role of the federal government have in curriculum design—the first steps having been taken in its specification of areas of research for the funding of training grants? Finally, how is the problem of maintaining innovation, academic growth, and faculty morale to be resolved in the face of worsening financial conditions?

SUMMARY

To summarize the major trends and developments of the last five years as discerned by the Macy Foundation survey:

- Little change in premedical admissions requirements;
- A decline in the importance of the MCAT, and a desire to utilize nonacademic criteria fairly in the selection of students;
- An overall increase in the number of applicants, as well as in their GPAs and MCAT scores;
- A sharp rise in the number of women students;
- An apparent leveling-off in the enrollment of minority group students;
- Students are more serious, goal-oriented, and concerned about the quality of medical care;
- Major curricular innovations have generally endured but are under scrutiny;
- A trend away from the three-year curriculum;
- A return to letter or numerical grading;
- Continuing interest in elective tracking, early clinical experience, and independent study programs; and
- Changes in the use of NMBE examinations.

Teaching the Biological Sciences
to Premedical Students

THOMAS B. ROOS

Education in biology, as in any other subject, changes in response to two sets of pressures. The first grows internally from added information and novel interpretation. The second derives from student needs and preparation, institutional organization, and social priorities.

Ten years ago, changes in biological education developed as biologists deepened and broadened their understanding of life processes, using new ways to look at nature and allowing cross-fertilization of ideas to occur between distinct scientific disciplines. Excitement and change triggered by research coincided with external demands for university expansion to accommodate more students, new kinds of students, and new programs. Many traditional departments were transformed, and facilities were enlarged.

Societal interest was reflected tangibly in monetary largesse. Support for scientific research, application, and education abounded from both public and private sources. Faith in the continuation of such affluence attracted many students to careers in science, without reducing the numbers entering applied fields.

Biology moved rapidly away from the review of plant and animal life, comparative morphology, and organ physiology, which had dominated teaching and thought since the time of Huxley and Haeckel, grounding itself more firmly in genetics, the physical sciences, and mathematics. Taxonomic distinctions gave way to organizational ones, systematics transmuted itself into system analysis. Where once all biology was divided into either botany and zoology, it has reordered itself systematically, recognizing five kingdoms (Monera, Protista, planta, fungi, and animalia), and analytically by levels of organization (molecular, cellular, organismal, populational, or societal) (Figure 1). Whereas the terms physiologist, anatomist, and geneticist once sufficed to characterize differences in approach among biologists, such new distinctions as biochemist, molecular biologist, cytologist, ecologist, ethologist, developmental biologist, and immunologist appeared almost as fast as the words could be coined.

Increasing fundamental knowledge and intellectual activity produced courses quite different from those known to Abraham Flexner, on which most medical educators still base their ideas of a proper premedical background. The release from old thought habits, in turn, stimulated biologists to undertake new kinds of research, opening up investigations of areas that had previously been considered out of bounds: social organization; perception and learning; language and communication; information theory; and energy transduction. Recycled, this knowledge fits comfortably into the new framework, contributing to its richness, but extending the time required to teach it and accelerating its development. The internal force toward change thus continues to operate, despite a decade of active response.

EXTERNAL PRESSURES

External pressures on biological education, for both prospective biologists and physicians, have since 1965 resulted from forces less sanguine than those of the previous decade. Student aspirations and attitudes have changed. Economic stringency has imposed itself on both education and career planning. A revolution in university administration has brought strange, often bizarre, notions of efficiency, accountability, and equivalency into the institution, in company with a flood of new academic managers. Academic freedom and scholarship have been denigrated and endangered by the application of management techniques and models of corporate organization. Graduate study, once an attractive option, has become a costly preparation for an uncertain future.

By attracting potential research-oriented scientists, the financial rewards of medicine act to society's detriment, filling scarce admissions places with people who are not interested in primary care. The medical degree does, however, protect against dwindling research support, elimination of faculty positions, and poor financial compensation. Even young faculty members in biology departments

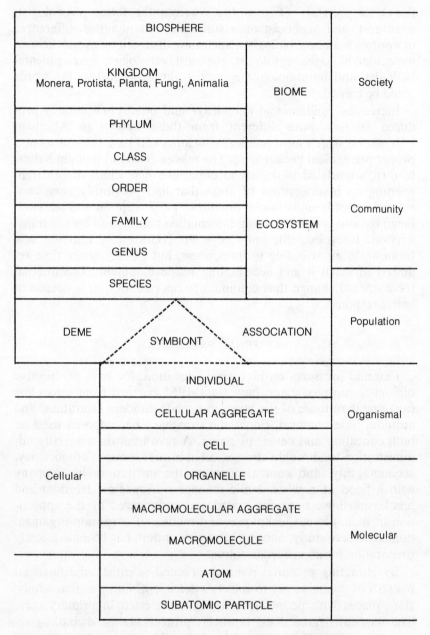

Figure 1. Hierarchical Organization of Biological Systems.

have given up writing letters of recommendation for others, in favor of submitting their own applications.

Increased competition for admission, especially from academically strong candidates, has brought about a state of affairs that was common in the postwar period, but happily reduced during the 1960s. Success in the competition for admission to medical school too often goes to those more interested in being a doctor than in practicing humane medicine. Although ambition, whether for status, wealth, or fame, need neither preclude compassion or forbid practicing community or family medicine in rural or inner city areas, it is more likely to lead to a medical center post or to a suburban practice. The intense competition and unpredictable criteria for success have, moreover, provoked cynicism, even among premedical students who seemed largely immune to recent, pandemic political disillusionment. Cynicism has in turn given rise to a pervasive lack of interest in course content and to a concern for grades. Both are bad in themselves, but worse for their contribution to the consumerization of higher education.

INTERNAL PRESSURES

Intense student desire to attend medical school might seem to benefit biology departments, since it multiplies the number of students enrolled in biology courses and thus strengthens the department's position in the budgetary sweepstakes. Numerical increase has, however, come at a difficult time in the life of American universities. The combination of economic exigency and managerial reorganization has prevented hiring new faculty members, even in departments with large enrollments, such as biology. It has simultaneously provided administrative justification for decreasing the number of faculty in those subjects abandoned by students in their rush toward medicine.

Moreover, high costs associated with teaching biology laboratory courses and supporting faculty investigations have increased the demands on existing space and equipment, have interfered with their replacement, and have thus curtailed course improvement. These factors have particularly affected large courses elected by premedical students, which often constitute their only experience in science. Higher enrollments also increase the amount of time spent by faculty members in advising, tutoring, and writing recommendations, as well as in course administration. The burden is made especially grievous by the decline in the numbers of students who intend to pursue academic or research careers. As a recent issue of the *Harvard Crimson* stated, to choose a biology major "is a euphemism for wanting to become a doctor."

Many biology departments have responded with a seeming paradox: they are increasing the number of introductory courses offered in canned format, that is, audio-tutorial or the Keller plan, of advanced courses offered for independent study, or of project-oriented, rather than didactic, experiences. This has simultaneously diminished the experimental, questing nature of the initial courses, while throwing students on their own into advanced courses with inadequate preparation. While the greater freedom to do research has satisfied a desire among students for a more direct involvement in their own education, it has also excused the imposition of restrictions on class size and made many courses less accessible.

As with any attempt to resolve a paradox, the results are uneven. Larger numbers of students learn about science instead of doing science. They are accommodated in beginning courses, and encouraged in advanced ones, to substitute "learning experiences" for scholarship. On the positive side, early opportunities for research do stimulate interest, generate participation, and establish a kind of independence; on the negative side, they encourage superficial, spotty learning and hubris. Whether good or bad, however, research experience is no longer unusual among undergraduates; it forms an integral part of most college biology programs.

The combined premedical-biological surge has propagated its effects throughout the university. For teachers of college undergraduates these are indeed "interesting times," in the full sense of the Chinese curse. Parabiological courses have burgeoned, capitalizing on the desire of students to impress admissions committees with their sincerity in pursuing medical careers, and of departments to swell their enrollments.

The basis for planning and grading many of these courses reflects the influence of managerial thinking that regards students as "products," whose quality is measured by acceptance into corporations or professional schools. Indeed, college recruiters use their institution's record of "success" in placement as a lure to prospective applicants. Internal pressures grow to inflate grades and produce complimentary letters of recommendation in order to improve the college's "score," which erodes honest judgment and evaluation. These tendencies increase with the proportion of professional managers in administrative posts. Clearly not all pressures to change are desirable, and not all "recent changes in teaching . . ." are progressive.

COLLEGE SUPPLIERS OF MEDICAL STUDENTS

Approximately two thousand American colleges grant the baccalaureate degree, but only a few send significant numbers of their graduates to medical school (Table 1). The majority of entrants will have prepared at one of a small number of colleges, mostly units of large universities with integral medical schools, whose total enrollments exceed ten thousand. Approximately 60 percent of all first-year medical students attend only about one hundred colleges.

Although nearly twice as many individuals enter medical school now as in 1960, there has been little change in their collegiate origins.[1, 2] A trend toward greater diversity in undergraduate background appeared between 1960 and 1965, but quickly stabilized itself. Thus, in the 1950s, 31 percent of the sixty-one hundred students who entered first-year classes came from just twenty-five colleges.[3] By 1966 the first twenty-five colleges supplied only 28 percent of the eighty-seven hundred persons in freshmen classes.[4] The same percentage of the approximately eleven thousand students who entered in 1973 also came from the top twenty-five colleges.[5]

A new factor has further decreased diversity in recent years, as some medical schools have undertaken special combined programs in which students can proceed directly from high school through to the award of the M.D. degree in a shorter period of time. All of these schools are in universities whose undergraduate colleges are among the "top twenty-five." Expanding the list to include the thirty major college sources of medical students in 1973, only one was in a university with a total enrollment below five thousand; only one had no medical school in direct association; only one had a population of upperclassmen smaller than two thousand; and only one had a faculty size of less than five hundred. Almost all are located in urban centers. Twenty-three schools on the list (77 percent) were also among the top thirty in the 1950s. Most of the new ones are in the Northeast and Midwest, while those they replaced are in the South. The small cities once surrounding these colleges have become large metropolises. Preparation for medical school has thus become increasingly associated with large, northern, urban colleges, quite different in spirit from their predecessors.

TABLE 1. THIRTY COLLEGES IN THE UNITED STATES THAT SUPPLIED MOST MEDICAL STUDENTS IN 1973, COMPARED TO THEIR STATUS IN EARLIER YEARS

School	Rank			University Enrollment		Graduates Entering Medical School	
	1973	1966	1950s	Total	Upper Division	1973	1950–59 Average
Brown	14	*	*	6,000	2,000	131	22
California, Berkeley	7	5	7	28,000	11,000	170	90
Los Angeles	20	21	30	27,000	10,000	111	47
Columbia	28	8	5	14,000	2,000	94	98
Cornell	12	4	16	16,000	3,000	148	68
Dartmouth	27	7	25	4,000	2,000	94	52
Duke	24	*	23	9,000	2,000	100	57
Emory	29	19	12	6,000	2,000	93	74
Florida	30	*	*	20,000	9,000	92	22
Harvard	2	1	1	23,000	3,000	262	136
Illinois, Urbana	11	6	4	32,000	12,000	155	99
Indiana, Bloomington	8	9	10	68,000	10,000	166	84
Johns Hopkins	17	22	*	9,000	1,000	120	35
Kansas	21	*	19	19,000	7,000	105	60
Massachusetts Institute of Technology	15	*	*	7,000	2,000	127	9
Michigan	1	2	2	41,000	10,000	283	127
Michigan State	16	*	*	41,000	17,000	123	19
Minnesota	13	17	6	45,000	13,000	134	91

North Carolina	26	*	21	20,000	4,000	97	58
Northwestern	10	12	29	14,000	3,000	163	48
Notre Dame	22	11	*	8,000	3,000	178	63
Ohio State	23	15	13	45,000	16,000	102	74
Pennsylvania	5	13	17	17,000	3,000	178	63
Pennsylvania State	19	24	*	52,000	14,000	114	30
Princeton	18	14	18	6,000	2,000	118	61
Stanford	3	10	14	11,000	3,000	227	73
Texas, Austin	6	16	8	40,000	15,000	172	89
Vanderbilt	25	*	25	6,000	2,000	99	52
Wisconsin, Madison	9	18	9	34,000	13,000	164	85
Yale	4	3	11	10,000	2,000	205	77
Alabama	*	*	24	13,000	5,000	52	55
City College of New York	*	20	54	21,000	6,000	67	33
Iowa	*	*	22	19,000	7,000	74	57
Louisiana State	*	23	32	43,000	8,000	63	46
New York University	*	*	3	40,000	5,000	63	117
Pittsburgh	*	25	15	26,000	7,000	65	70
Tennessee	*	*	27	27,000	8,000	61	50
Tulane	*	*	20	9,000	2,000	77	60
Washington	*	*	27	31,000	12,000	88	50

Source: The above table has been compiled from information, recomputed and rearranged, in: "Datagram: Undergraduate Origins of Medical Students," Journal of Medical Education 44, no. 8 (1969): 712–13; W. F. Dubé, "Datagram: Undergraduate Origins of U.S. Medical Students," Journal of Medical Education 49, no. 10 (1974): 1005–10; William A. Manuel and Marion A. Altenderfer, Baccalaureate Origins of 1950–59 Medical Graduates, Public Health Monograph No. 66 (Washington: U.S. Government Printing Office, 1962); and Davis G. Johnson, Vernon C. Smith, Jr., and Stephen L. Tarnoff, "Recruitment and Progress of Minority Medical School Entrants 1970–72," Journal of Medical Education 50, no. 7 (1975): 713–55.
* Not among the first thirty.

Since more than half of medical school entrants major in biology,[6] and since so many prospective medical students prepare at so few colleges, it seemed sensible to restrict this survey to biology courses and programs at the thirty principal supplier-colleges. Twenty-four were selected on the simple criterion that their catalogues were both available and lucid.

Each college offers biology to its students in a unique format, often with optional paths toward a biology major and without apparent uniformity in basic instruction. At least one hundred different and acceptable routes can be plotted from the published descriptions of these twenty-four schools; greater familiarity with the realities of waivers, unwritten options, and so on, would most likely yield still more.

Not only the major program but individual course descriptions, including that for the initial course, differ markedly from school to school. Thus the admonition that premedical students should present "a year of biology with laboratory" when seeking acceptance to medical school is without real meaning. In some schools that requirement can be satisfied by courses that would have been familiar to Flexner or to the oldest living medical educator. At others, the prescribed year may itself require preparation by the student in mathematics, chemistry, and physics beyond the basic premedical levels. With diligence and the proper catalogue a student could select courses with suitable titles in which either nothing larger than a cell or smaller than a population appeared. Most schools offer an introductory course, however, based on biological principles. These courses may last only one quarter, or they may extend throughout an entire year. Some schools, on the other hand, have dispensed entirely with an introductory course.

Several colleges present their basic material in the form of a "core program" that may last two or even three years. In such programs, cell biology, genetics, anatomy, and embryology may be totally subsumed, separate courses with these titles appearing only at advanced levels. A beginning course in genetics, for example, appears in only eighteen catalogues, and one in cell biology in twenty; one school offers a single course in which genetics and cell biology are taught together. Comparative anatomy appears as a separate course in fifteen catalogues; embryology (or developmental biology) in seventeen; and a combined anatomy-embryology course in six others.

The programs surveyed in 1975 reflect changes made prior to 1965. Exhaustive studies carried out five to ten years ago under the aegis of the Commission on Undergraduate Education in the Biological Sciences (CUEBS) revealed no single format, text, or set of courses common among college biology departments.[7, 8] Despite their difference in order of presentation and course arrangement, however, all departments presented 75 percent of similar, and only 25 percent of idiosyncratic, material to their majors throughout the program, taken as a whole. The common 75 percent can be taken to represent "core knowledge: basic to any further study related to biology." The CUEBS panel that examined the education of biology majors concluded, among other things, that

. . . approximately two years is needed to communicate information commonly required in all biological specialties . . . [and that] titles and contents of courses vary widely and depart considerably from traditional biology courses. . . . There is a general departure from earlier curricula in placing greater emphasis on molecular, cellular, and population biology at the expense of . . . [all but] the developmental and physiological aspects of organismal biology. . ." [9]

Individual differences in packaging probably have no greater influence on the content of a major in 1975 than in 1965, and profoundly affect the kind of knowledge available to students who have taken only one or two courses in the major. Since these students may account for as many as half the medical school entrants in a given year,[10] half of each first-year class may have serious deficiencies.

Another CUEBS study panel explored those aspects of biology deemed most important in premedical preparation by medical school faculty members.[11] The subject areas most often identified as desirable largely reflected the traditional "premed" constellation: comparative anatomy, embryology, organ physiology, and what might be called classical vertebrate zoology; to this were added genetics, cell biology, behavior, and some aspects of ecology. Although each subject would appear in an introductory course, none could be covered in sufficient depth to give students a working knowledge in just one year. The study group, which was composed of individuals active in postbaccalaureate medical and health-related education, as well as biologists from undergraduate colleges, concluded:

Preparation for practice in any of the health sciences must include a theoretical background in biology equivalent to that in a biology core program. . . . Satisfactory performance in a rigorous course is preferable to a trival one. Special courses designed only to prepare students for professional study are inadequate.[12]

Accepting the theses that biological preparation is necessary for medicine and that special premedical courses are undesirable, and, further, given the extreme variation in content distribution in the undergraduate programs, one calendar year of biology is clearly insufficient to produce suitable biological literacy. Contrast this with the existing requirements for admission to medical school: one year in ninety-three schools (82 percent); one and one half in twelve (11 percent); and two in only eight (7 percent). One school that accepts students only from high school has no college biology requirement. Moreover, many accept high school advanced placement credits in lieu of a college course. Clearly, medical schools have perpetuated a myth of a scientific basis to medicine without insisting on its truth in practice. The prospect is a reversion of medical education into mere technical training.

CURRENT PRESSURES

The thoughts expressed in this paper stem from reflection on the degree to which science has been downgraded in medical education, and on how even old changes in biological education have been ignored by the medical schools. Current pressures to alter the nature of liberal education and its relation to the traditional learned professions are being exerted by anti-intellectual forces active both in society at large and within the universities. Not the least of these are the advocates of free-enterprise medicine, who neglect the scientific precepts of Hippocrates for the mysteries of the shaman and the economics of the entrepreneur, who would limit admissions, and who oppose meaningful alternatives to a medical career. Too many students wise enough to prepare for the study of medicine find themselves either excluded from the profession and unable to use their knowledge or enrolled in schools that disregard their knowledge.

Biological knowledge has continued to expand in areas foreign to the experience of many medical educators. Although molecular biology has been placed safely inside the pale of the preclinical years, sociobiology, ecology, population genetics, and developmental biology remain largely ignored. Too many physicians forget the lessons of science in their uncritical acceptance of the puffery of pharmaceutical advertising, of health faddists, or of pseudoscientific promoters. They endanger their patients in the process. A strong dose of scientific skepticism might protect against such gullibility, but only if the basic sciences, biology in particular, are studied free of the cynical attitudes induced by present admissions policies.

Perhaps it is time to consider some alternatives: one would abandon the pretense of a scientific base to modern medicine, allowing apprenticeships to replace costly medical schools; the other would accept the importance of science in preparation for medicine, revise existing, outdated requirements, and offer either open enrollment to any student who satisfied an established set of new requirements, or select a smaller number from among this group by lot instead of by artificial, always subjective, and often specious criteria.

Notes

1. "Datagram: Undergraduate Origins of Medical Students," *Journal of Medical Education* 44, no. 8 (1969): 712–13.

2. W. F. Dubé, "Datagram: Undergraduate Origins of U.S. Medical Students," *Journal of Medical Education* 49, no. 10 (1974): 1005–10.

3. William A. Manuel and Marion A. Altenderfer, *Baccalaureate Origins of 1950–59 Medical Graduates,* Public Health Monograph No. 66 (Washington: U.S. Government Printing Office, 1962).

4. "Origins of Medical Students" (see note 1).

5. Dubé, "Origins of U.S. Medical Students" (see note 2).

6. Davis G. Johnson, Vernon C. Smith, Jr., and Stephen L. Tarnoff, "Recruitment and Progress of Minority Medical School Entrants 1970–72," *Journal of Medical Education* 50, no. 7 (1975): 713–55, especially tables on pp. 745–55.

7. Commission on Undergraduate Education in the Biomedical Sciences, *Content of Core Curricula in Biology,* CUEBS Publication No. 18 (Washington: Commission on Undergraduate Education in Biomedical Sciences, 1967).

8. Donald D. Cox and Lary V. Davis, *The Context of Biological Education: The Case for Change,* CUEBS Publication No. 34, Appendix A (Washington: Commission on Undergraduate Education in the Biomedical Sciences, 1972): 121–26.

9. Commission on Biomedical Sciences, *Core Curricula in Biology* (see note 7).

10. Johnson, Smith, and Tarnoff, "Minority Medical School Entrants" (see note 6).

11. Thomas B. Roos, *Biological Prerequisites for Education in the Health Sciences,* CUEBS Publication No. 27 (Washington: Commission on Undergraduate Education in the Biomedical Sciences, 1969).

12. Ibid.

DISCUSSION

It was pointed out that some of the colleges listed in Roos's table preselect students for whom they will write recommendations for medical school, while others will consider anyone who wishes to be a premedical student. The first group of schools will naturally have a higher proportion of students admitted to medical school, regardless of their overall class sizes.

The drifting apart of the arts and science faculties and their medical school counterparts is seen as a major problem. Students perceive the differences between the two, in that, for example, some faculty members must work longer hours than others and "hustle" for grant support. This latter situation—the disparity in the levels of grant support—is a major cause of envy and dissention.

There is at the present time intense pressure in the universities to reduce the sizes of departments whose enrollments are down. While this may not be a great problem in, say, an English department with forty faculty members, it is a real threat to a religion department if it loses two of its total of five teachers. The question is: Can a university education be efficient? The answer is: No.

The discussion turned to the quality of biology preparation for medical school. Because only one year of biology is required by most medical schools, there is a great variability in the quality of preparation—a variability that does not exist in the physical sciences, where there is uniformity in the length and content of the courses required.

Participants felt that a special premedical course, the desirability of which is questionable at best, would have to be designed in order to do a proper job of biology preparation in one year. On the other hand, merely lengthening the time required, that is, to make two years the norm, is not the answer, because a large variety of courses are offered under the heading, "biology." What is needed is a specification of the requirements, as is the case in the physical sciences, that is, five hours each of inorganic, organic, and physical chemistry.

In conclusion it was felt that two years of preparation in biology is desirable. A greater emphasis on quantitative biology, based on molecular and cellular concepts, is essential.

The Admissions Process

JOSEPH CEITHAML

I shall first describe the actual admissions process in medical schools in the United States, and then discuss several factors that have had significant impact on that process. In recent years the medical school selection process has undergone an appreciable number of refinements and modifications. The objective of the process remains essentially unaltered, however: to select the best qualified applicants for the entering classes. Some of the changes in the selection process have evolved by design, others have been imposed by circumstances.

Basically, in the selection of medical students, admissions committees first focus their attention on the intellectual abilities of each applicant; if he * qualifies in this regard, then and only then do the committees consider the equally important, but much more elusive, nonintellective characteristics. This in no way implies that admissions committees consider intellectual ability more important than any other qualities. There is a sound rationale for this initial screening of medical applicants, for if they are not intellectually capable of coping successfully with a rigorous program of medical studies, no matter how honest, forthright, personable, and otherwise desirable they may be, they will never become physicians. On the other hand, sufficient intelligence and acceptable scholastic achievement alone do not automatically qualify an individual for admission. Consequently, various nonintellective qualities are carefully considered before a scholastically qualified applicant is offered a place in a medical school class.

When a student applies to a medical school he is usually asked to submit the following credentials: 1) one or two application forms; 2) a transcript of his college grades; 3) his Medical College Admis-

---

* Throughout this paper the terms "he," "his," and "him" are used generically to include "she" and "her."

sion Test (MCAT) scores; and 4) premedical advisory reports from his undergraduate college.

INTELLECTUAL CHARACTERISTICS

In reviewing a student's college record, admissions committees consider not only his grades, but the college he has attended, for it is recognized that academic standards vary from one school to another; at some, high grades are more difficult to achieve than in others. It is on the basis of their past experience with students from different colleges that the committees have become aware of these factors.

Unfortunately, in recent years the task of evaluating academic records has been made more difficult. Grades, in general, have been inflated; unsatisfactory and failing grades at some colleges are not recorded on the academic records; and the grade point averages (GPAs) have generally risen appreciably. This grade inflation has occurred widely among colleges, even the most prestigious of them. It is reported that the average GPA of students at one highly regarded college is 3.5 and rising; one of the reasons given for this is that the school has discontinued using D and F grades. At another prestigious college, in the academic year 1974–75 over 80 percent of all grades were As or Bs.

In appraising an applicant's intellectual ability on the basis of his college academic record, admissions committees also consider the effort expended by the student in compiling his grade average. If he carries a heavy academic program of study, including one or more time-consuming and demanding laboratory courses, he is less likely to receive high grades than if he carries a light schedule of courses. Similarly, the committees appreciate the fact that, among applicants from the same college, the same GPA may represent little effort on the part of one student and supreme effort on the part of another. The former student might be expected to possess a reserve of academic strength that the latter does not, which could mean the difference between success and failure in medical school.

It is in this regard, therefore, that the committees turn to the candidate's record of extracurricular interests and part-time work activities. A student who is a member of an athletic team, the school newspaper staff, or student government may spend many hours each week in these pursuits. On the other hand, the student who serves as a laboratory or research assistant, or the one who finds it necessary to work part time to help finance his education, each devotes a considerable amount of time to these activities. It is evident that such students could have compiled better GPAs if they had devoted to their studies the time expended on their extracurricular undertakings. The committees take cognizance of this in their evaluation of the applicant's academic achievements.

In addition to the student's official academic record, to a greater or lesser extent many medical schools utilize the MCAT scores in evaluating students' intellectual capabilities. It should be noted immediately, however, that most admissions committees put much less emphasis on MCAT scores than is generally thought to be the case. The MCAT is a three-hour, objective-type test consisting of four subtests:

1. *Verbal Ability:* A measure of vocabulary strength and ability to perceive verbal relationships.

2. *Quantitative Ability:* A measure of ability to reason through and understand quantitative concepts and relationships.

3. *General Information:* A measure of factual knowledge in non-science fields, including art, economics, geography, government, history, literature, music, philosophy, and psychology.

4. *Science:* A measure of factual knowledge in science, including a wide sampling of concepts and problems taken from basic college courses in biology, chemistry, and physics.

Most medical schools in the United States require applicants to take the MCAT, for it gives them a means of comparing the performance of students from different colleges on the same test. In cases where an applicant has a good college GPA and high MCAT scores, or, conversely, a poor college record and low MCAT scores, admissions committees of most medical schools have no problem in reaching a decision. The former candidate qualifies on scholastic grounds; the latter does not.

On the other hand, problems arise when there are inconsistencies between the college grades and the MCAT scores. Low MCAT scores coupled with a high GPA may mean that the college in question has an easy grading system, or that the student, by concentrating solely on his studies and by dint of great effort on his part, was able to achieve good grades despite limited intellectual capacity. In such a case it would be questionable whether the applicant has sufficient ability to complete a demanding program of medical studies successfully. High MCAT scores coupled with a low GPA may suggest that the applicant has intellectual potentialities that he has not utilized effectively in his studies. Such an underachiever may have considerable promise as a medical student, provided the interfering factors can be remedied or eliminated. In any event, whenever a committee is faced with discrepancies between an applicant's college academic record and his MCAT scores, it must investigate further to determine the reasons for the discrepancies before assessing the applicant's intellectual qualities.

In this regard, letters written on behalf of the applicant by his premedical advisor or premedical committee chairman and his instructors at college frequently will contain pertinent information. Such letters are most helpful to a committee in reaching a decision.

NONINTELLECTIVE CHARACTERISTICS

Once it has been established that an applicant possesses the necessary qualifications to study medicine, the admissions committee turns its attention to the nonintellective characteristics of this scholastically acceptable applicant. Such characteristics as integrity, initiative, character, emotional stability, motivation, and determinaton are all very highly regarded by committee members. It is recognized, however, that these are very difficult to assess. As might be expected, the task of evaluating the personality and character of medical applicants is approached by different medical schools in a variety of ways. In general, four main sources of information are considered, usually in the following manner: 1) the application form itself; 2) premedical advisory reports from the undergraduate college; 3) personal interviews; and 4) psychological tests.

Medical school application forms include a wide variety of questions, and, in addition, usually request a written essay or autobiographical sketch intended to secure information regarding the nonintellective characteristics of the applicant. Such information in the completed forms is usually superficial or merely suggestive, however; much more meaningful information can be obtained from other sources.

The student's premedical advisory report often plays an important role in the evaluation of his nonintellective characteristics. Frequently such a report consists not only of a letter from the premedical committee or premedical advisor, but of individual letters from instructors, and occasionally a letter from the student's dormitory head resident. It is generally agreed by committee members that at the present time the premedical advisory report is perhaps the best source for appraising an applicant's character, integrity, and leadership qualities. Moreover, they appreciate the fact that it is highly desirable to maintain good rapport with the premedical advisory groups at the colleges their applicants attend in order to ensure candor and completeness in the reports. This is especially true in light of the Buckley Amendment to the Family Educational Rights and Privacy Act of 1974.

If at this point in the selection procedure the committee is impressed by the student's credentials it will usually invite him for a personal interview, either at the medical school or, if it is too far distant, locally with a representative of the medical school. The interview is a widely used technique for obtaining information about the nonintellective characteristics of applicants. It should be added, however, that there is a considerable difference of opinion as to its value in the selection process. In most medical schools the interview is not used to predict scholastic success, but to fill a variety of other purposes. For example, it allows the student an opportunity to explain in person any unique or complicated aspects of his application. At the same time it affords the admissions committee an opportunity to verify or clarify information obtained from the application form and from other sources.

The interview may also be used to detect gross deficiencies in the personality and emotional stability of an applicant. In cases where emotional problems become a consideration, the student is usually referred to a psychiatrist for an extensive interview. Currently, many medical schools regard the interview as a two-way process—the school gets an opportunity to become acquainted with the student, and he is given a chance to learn more about the school to which he has applied.

At most medical schools, after the interview report has been considered in conjunction with all other pertinent information, the admissions committee makes its decision and notifies the applicant. At some schools, however, one or more psychological tests may be administered to prospective candidates before a final decision is reached. Usually referred to as personality and vocational interest tests, they include measures of interpersonal relations, personal values, interests, attitudes, and personal adjustment. Many questions are currently being raised as to the reliability of these psychological tests and the validity of the scores—questions that must be resolved before the tests can be widely used with confidence in selecting medical students. Nevertheless, such tests do show promise, and an Association of American Medical Colleges (AAMC) task force on the Medical College Admissions Assessment Program (MCAAP) is working diligently in that direction.

Thus far I have described the general procedures employed by an admissions committee in selecting the best possible candidates from each medical school's pool of applicants. These procedures appear to have been successful in identifying individuals who can and do complete their medical studies satisfactorily; consistently in recent years about 95 percent of all students embarking on a program of medical studies ultimately graduate and receive their M.D. degrees.[1]

FACTORS AFFECTING THE ADMISSIONS PROCESS

At the outset of this paper it was noted that the selection process has undergone refinements and changes. It is desirable to explore the nature of these changes—what may have prompted them, and their effect on the selection process. Probably the single most important factor affecting the admissions process today is the dramatic rise in the ratio of applicants to places available in entering medical classes [2,3] (Table 1). During the past fifteen years there has been almost a 75 percent increase in first-year places. In this same span of time, however, the number of medical school *applicants* each year has almost tripled, while the number of *applications* submitted has increased fivefold: medical school admissions committees have been inundated with applications. In 1972, twenty-one schools each received over five thousand applications; five of these schools actually had an excess of eight thousand applications for their entering classes. There has, incidentally, been a much sharper rise in the number of female applicants than male applicants, as can be seen in Table 2.[4] Similarly, the number of applications from minority group students has grown steadily.[5]

MATCHING PLAN

To cope with the flood of applications, from time to time it has been suggested that a matching plan be instituted for the selection of medical students. Proponents of this notion have pointed to the eminently successful National Internship and Residency Matching Program (NIRMP), by which graduating medical students secure

TABLE 1. SUMMARY OF UNITED STATES MEDICAL SCHOOL APPLICANTS AND FIRST-YEAR ENROLLEES

First-Year Class	Number of Schools	Number of Applicants (1)	Number of Applications (2)	Ratio of Applications to Applicant (2) ÷ (1)	First-Year Enrollment (3)	Ratio of Applicants to First-Year Places (3) ÷ (1)
1958–59	85	15,170	59,102	3.9	8,128	1.9
1961–62	87	14,381	53,834	3.7	8,483	1.7
1963–64	87	17,668	70,063	4.0	8,772	2.0
1968–69	99	21,112	112,195	5.3	9,863	2.1
1969–70	101	24,465	133,822	5.5	10,422	2.4
1970–71	103	24,987	148,797	6.0	11,348	2.2
1971–72	108	29,172	210,943	7.2	12,361	2.4
1972–73	112	36,135	267,306	7.4	13,677	2.6
1973–74	114	40,506	328,275	8.1	14,124	2.9

Source: W. F. Dubé and D. G. Johnson, "Study of U.S. Medical Applicants, 1973–74," *Journal of Medical Education* 50, no. 11 (1975); 1015–33; and Anne E. Crowley, ed., "Medical Education in the United States, 1973–74," *Journal of the American Medical Association*, suppl. 231 (January 1975): 1–139.

TABLE 2. SUMMARY OF UNITED STATES MEDICAL SCHOOL APPLICANTS
AND FIRST-YEAR ENROLLEES BY SEX

First-Year Class	Applicants			First-Year Enrollees		
	Number of Men	Number of Women	Percentage of Women	Number of Men	Number of Women	Percentage of Women
1970–71	22,253	2,734	10.9	10,092	1,256	11.1
1971–72	25,435	3,737	12.8	10,668	1,693	13.7
1972–73	30,655	5,480	15.1	11,377	2,300	16.8
1973–74	33,304	7,202	17.8	11,338	2,786	19.7
1974–75	33,912	8,712	20.4	11,488	3,275	22.2

Source: W. F. Dubé, "Datagram: U.S. Medical Student Enrollment 1970–71
Through 1974–75," *Journal of Medical Education* 50, no. 3 (1975): 303–06.

their first-year postgraduate clinical appointments. Consequently,
for the 1974 entering classes the AAMC conducted two, concurrent,
pilot medical school matching programs. One involved the eight
medical schools located in California; the other, the three medical
schools in Michigan. The rationale for these two specific programs
was that applicants to the Michigan medical schools usually apply
to all three, and that, similarly, applicants to the California schools,
especially state residents, often apply to most, if not all eight.

There is, however, a basic and important difference between the
NIRMP and a medical school matching program. The NIRMP
represents a "buyer's market," while the latter corresponds to a
"seller's market": there are many more first-year postgraduate clinical appointment positions available annually in the United States
than there are graduating students; on the other hand, there are
about three medical school applicants for each available place in
entering classes. A medical school matching plan would therefore
greatly increase the work of admissions committees. Since the medical schools would not know until the time of matching which of the
acceptable applicants would actually take the offered places, the
committees would have to consider many more applicants than they
do now. This would necessitate a greater number of interviews,
which would create additional work for the committees and require
the expenditure of extra time and more money by the applicants.

With the present rolling admissions procedure, as students are
selected by medical schools they withdraw their applications for
further consideration by schools lower on their lists. In this way
committees are spared the necessity of considering applicants who

intend to enroll elsewhere. It is not surprising, therefore, that after the AAMC pilot matching programs were completed it was concluded that it was not feasible to implement the plan for medical students at the present time.

EARLY DECISION PLAN

A much better way to reduce the numbers of applications processed by admissions committees is the early decision plan (EDP), whereby a student may request and receive an early decision on his application to the medical school of his first choice, prior to applying elsewhere. He is obliged to submit all his admissions material—application forms, academic record, MCAT scores, and letters of recommendation—to the medical school of his first choice by August 15; the school in turn agrees to make a decision by October 1.

One of three decisions may be rendered: the applicant may be accepted, and thus need not apply elsewhere; he may be rejected, and subsequently may concentrate all his efforts on other medical schools; or, finally, if a school is unable to reach a decision by October 1 the applicant may be so notified and told that the school will consider him further in the regular competition involving non-EDP applicants. While such an applicant therefore still has a chance for acceptance by the medical school of his first choice, he may apply to other schools. Since the average number of applications per applicant now exceeds eight, for each individual accepted by an EDP seven others are, in essence, removed from the applicant pool.

Although individual medical schools have long used their own versions of informal early decision plans, it was not until 1970 that all the medical schools in Chicago cooperatively participated in a formally announced EDP. In 1973, however, through the concerted efforts of the AAMC's Group on Student Affairs and its Division of Student Studies, a total of fifty-one medical schools decided to engage in the formal EDP, most of them for the first time, for the class entering in 1974. Table 3 shows a summary of the results of the EDP. For the class entering in 1975, for example, fifty-nine schools selected 818 EDP enrollees from a total of 1,889 applications. This removed about fifty-seven hundred highly qualified applicants from the pool, and saved admissions committees a considerable amount of "busy work" that otherwise would have been entailed in processing

TABLE 3. UNITED STATES MEDICAL SCHOOLS WITH
EARLY DECISION PLANS (EDPs): APPLICANTS AND ENROLLEES

First-Year Class	1974–75	1975–76	1976–77
Medical schools with EDP	51	59	59
EDP applicants	1,719	1,889	—
EDP enrollees	628	818	—

Source: Data supplied by the Association of American Medical Colleges, Division of Student Studies.

the applications of high-quality students who would sooner or later be accepted by the schools of their first choice.

If only 10 percent of available places in current entering classes were filled by the EDP, some fifteen hundred qualified individuals would thereby be selected, and about ten thousand five hundred high-quality applications would be eliminated from the pool. This would not only represent a considerable saving of time for admissions committees, but would enable them to concentrate their energies on those applicants who would be more likely to attend their medical schools if offered the opportunity. Thus a beneficial by-product of the EDP would be the improvement of the overall selection process at each school.

Similarly, the highly qualified applicant who has selected the medical school of his first choice also benefits. If accepted by the EDP, he need apply to no other school, thus saving him time, energy, and money. Moreover, these students reap an important dividend, for they can then devote their attention during their final year in college to academic and extracurricular activities. It should also be noted that the EDP applicant who is not accepted still has plenty of time to apply to other schools.

The EDP also benefits the undergraduate colleges, since their premedical advisors or advisory committees need submit but one set of supporting letters for the successful EDP applicant. Having done that, they may concentrate their efforts on behalf of their students who have not participated in the EDP.

Incidentally, some state-supported medical schools that normally select a relatively small number of out-of-state students each year have given thought to requiring nonresidents to apply for admission only via the EDP. In this way, a school could select those nonresidents who have a special reason for wishing to attend that institution; at the same time this tactic would eliminate the vast majority of nonresidents who may be applying only to have yet another potentially viable application on record.

In short, the EDP is beneficial to the applicants, to the colleges, and to the medical schools. It actually accelerates the consideration of all applicants by eliminating the successful high-quality EDP applicants who would merit consideration by virtually any medical school to which they applied.

AMERICAN MEDICAL COLLEGE APPLICATION SERVICE

Another recent and most valuable aid to admissions committees is the American Medical College Application Service (AMCAS), a nonprofit, centralized application-processing service, based in Washington, D.C., for applicants to American medical schools. AMCAS, developed by medical school admissions officers to facilitate the application procedures, was organized under the auspices of the AAMC. It went into operation on a nation-wide basis for the classes entering in 1971. Since then, each year more and more schools have availed themselves of this service (Table 4), for it benefits the applicants, their undergraduate colleges, and the medical schools.

The applicant to an AMCAS-participating school profits by submitting only one set of application material, including official transcripts and MCAT scores. AMCAS collates this material, checks and evaluates the student's academic records, coordinates and replicates the data, and sends a copy to each AMCAS school to which the applicant wishes to apply. The undergraduate college benefits, since it is asked to provide a single transcript to AMCAS, instead of one to each medical school to which the student applies. The medical schools are aided, since not only do they receive complete and processed application material for each applicant, but they need

TABLE 4. NUMBER OF MEDICAL SCHOOLS IN THE UNITED STATES PARTICIPATING IN THE AMERICAN MEDICAL COLLEGE APPLICATION SERVICE (AMCAS)

First-Year Class	1971–72	1972–73	1973–74	1974–75	1975–76	1976–77
Medical schools	108	112	114	114	114	114
Medical schools with AMCAS	56	58	70	75	83	86

Source: Anne E. Crowley, ed., "Medical Education in the United States, 1973–74," *Journal of the American Medical Association*, suppl. 231 (January 1975): 1–139; and data supplied by the Association of American Medical Colleges, Division of Student Studies.

not employ personnel to evaluate the various academic transcripts they receive from the many different colleges the applicants attend. The time saved by the admissions committees can be used in expediting the admissions process and in devoting more attention to the student than to his application material.

One disadvantage of AMCAS is that the ease of application may encourage students to apply to more schools, thereby still further increasing the applicant pool. This is partially offset by a graduated application fee based on the number of AMCAS applications made. One of the purposes of introducing the EDP was, likewise, to reduce the total number of AMCAS applications submitted each year. In any event, AMCAS has been of great assistance to admissions committees by effectively reducing the time and the expense of the application procedure.

LAWSUITS

Whereas AMCAS has eased the work of medical school admissions committees, another rather recent development is causing them distress. A spate of real or threatened lawsuits is harassing them and adding to their difficulties. A recent survey conducted by the AAMC Division of Student Studies revealed that from 1971 to 1974 court cases involving applicants to thirteen medical schools were in progress or had been settled.[6] In addition, thirty-five other schools reported threats of court action, that is, the schools had been contacted by a lawyer acting on an applicant's behalf.

Table 5 shows a summary of these activities. Of the nineteen actual cases, two were resolved in favor of the plaintiff. Both were

TABLE 5. SUMMARY OF LAWSUITS INVOLVING UNITED STATES MEDICAL SCHOOL APPLICANTS, 1971–74

Nature of Allegation Against the Medical School	Actual Lawsuits	Threatened Lawsuits
Racial bias	8	25
Sex bias	3	8
Age	1	5
Residency	1	4
Health	1	0
Other, unspecified	5	21
	19	63

Source: "AAMC Division of Student Studies," *The Student Affairs Reporter* 4 (1975): 1–8.

argued concurrently against the same medical school, and related to its discouraging female parents of small children from applying to the school. One case of reverse discrimination involving a California medical school was decided against the school: the court concluded that granting preference to minority students "denies white persons an equal opportunity for admittance." At the same time, however, the court declined to order the admission of the plaintiff, finding that his contention that he would have been admitted had it not been for a special minority group program was not sustained by the evidence. The remaining sixteen suits were dismissed for technical reasons, decided in favor of the medical schools, or are still in progress. In any event, such lawsuits, or even threats thereof, add to the burdens of the admissions committees and require the expenditures of large amounts of time, effort, and, in some cases, money.

MEDICAL COLLEGE ADMISSIONS ASSESSMENT PROGRAM

Reference was made earlier to the AAMC's Medical College Admissions Assessment Program (MCAAP), which was initiated in 1972 in response to the growing concern of medical educators about the large numbers of qualified applicants not admitted to medical schools each year, and the impact of the selection process on the quality and availability of health care.

Criticism had been directed at the selection process, which relied heavily on GPAs, MCAT scores, and premedical advisory reports. Its detractors claimed that graduates of our medical schools, while technically competent, tend too frequently to lack the humanistic qualities desired in physicians. Various failings in our nation's health care delivery system have been blamed, rightly or wrongly, on the medical schools and on their student selection process.

The MCAAP was established to conduct a comprehensive examination of the admissions process, one objective being to develop new measures, and to improve those currently being used, for the assessment of medical school applicants.

One of the MCAAP's recommendations was to develop new tests of cognitive and noncognitive abilities. The term "cognitive characteristics," synonymous with "intellectual attributes," pertains to intellectual ability and academic achievement; the term "noncognitive characteristics," interchangeable with "nonintellectual attributes," refers to the individual's personality, level of maturity, interests, emotional stability, and values.

New tests to assess cognition now being developed to replace the present MCAT will be in the areas of reading comprehension, quantitative reasoning, biology, chemistry, and physics. The assessment of reading skills will involve the comprehension and analysis of material chosen from the social sciences, the basic sciences, and clinical medicine. The quantitative section will stress problem solving, with less emphasis on computational skills. Finally, separate tests in biology, chemistry, and physics are planned to permit a better evaluation of the applicant's knowledge in these three science areas. It is expected that these new tests will replace the MCAT by the spring of 1977.

At the same time the cognitive tests are being developed, a task force is studying and planning ways to evaluate noncognitive factors. Three primary areas of concern here are the organization of knowledge in meaningful ways for medical practice; skills in dealing with patients; and attitudes. The noncognitive characteristics to be considered include concern for human needs; sensitivity toward others; decision-making abilities; staying power; performance in interprofessional relations; and orientation to lifelong learning.

After the instruments to test these noncognitive factors have been developed, much time and attention will need to be devoted to validating them before they can be used. Understandably, no timetable has been established for the implementation of these tests.

SUMMARY

In processing record numbers of applications, the majority of medical schools currently employ the AMCAS to provide basic information about the applicants. Many schools now also employ the EDP to select, as the nucleus of their classes, a small but appreciable number of entering students who express an interest in attending those schools above all others. The MCAT is in the process of being replaced by the new cognitive tests of the MCAAP, while strenuous efforts are being expended to provide long-awaited and much-needed companion noncognitive tests.

Our medical school admissions committees are having a difficult time. Faced, on the one hand, with a surfeit of qualified applicants, exhorted to accept more women, more minority group applicants, and, in essence, more students, and plagued, on the other hand, either by threats of lawsuits or by actual, time-consuming suits alleging discrimination on a variety of grounds, or, in some cases, reverse discrimination, the committees are doing a heroic job and are being remarkably successful in selecting entering medical school classes. Committee members, however, more than any other group, realize that the process of selection is not perfect, and are constantly seeking ways to improve it. The anticipated MCAAP cognitive tests, and, even more, the noncognitive tests, promise to become important additions to the armamentarium of the beleaguered admissions committees of our medical schools.

Notes

1. D. G. Johnson and W. E. Sedlacek, "Retention by Sex and Race of 1968–72 U.S. Medical School Entrants," *Journal of Medical Education* 50, no. 10 (1975): 925–33.
2. W. F. Dubé and D. G. Johnson, "Study of U.S. Medical Applicants, 1973–74," ibid., no. 11: 1015–33.
3. Anne E. Crowley, ed., "Medical Education in the United States, 1973–74," *Journal of the American Medical Association,* suppl. 231 (January 1975): 1–139.
4. W. F. Dubé, "Datagram. U.S. Medical Student Enrollment, 1970–71 Through 1974–75," *Journal of Medical Education* 50, no. 3 (1975): 303–06.
5. Dubé and Johnson, "Medical Applicants, 1973–74" (see note 2).
6. "AAMC Division of Student Studies," *The Student Affairs Reporter* 4 (1975): 1–8.

DISCUSSION

The identification of "noncognitive variables," that is, the proper assessment of qualities such as motivation and dedication, is a complex issue facing medical school admissions committees. The AAMC, the National Board of Medical Examiners, and the Educational Testing Service are actively engaged in research in this area, as are groups at the universities of Minnesota and Iowa.

Regarding the make-up of the admissions committees, a one-person "committee" was cited by some of the discussants as more likely to take chances than a large committee, which will usually opt for the mean, in other words, the safe. Nonetheless, the practicality and general desirability of a one-man committee was questioned, except when the services of a uniquely qualified and committed individual are available.

The series of lawsuits being brought against admissions committees by unsuccessful applicants was discussed. A number of medical schools have legal advisors in the dean's office; one dean noted that he had three lawyers on his staff. It was felt that large admissions committees are no protection against legal actions. In fact, they merely provide more defendants. For the most part, admissions committees do not select students in their own images, and the conclusion was reached that committees should not be restructured because of threats of legal action.

The Medical Student, 1975

DAVIS G. JOHNSON

In spite of all the other significant trends that have taken place during the past few years, I believe most of us would agree that perhaps the most important single ingredient in determining the success of medical education is the caliber of the individual medical student.

I plan to approach the topic from three major vantage points: 1) by summarizing available statistics about recent changes in medical students; 2) by reporting subjective impressions of today's students from colleagues at the Association of American Medical Colleges (AAMC) and at representative medical schools; * and 3) by comparing contemporary national medical student organizations with their activities in the past. Although these findings, in general, demonstrate that our present medical student body is larger, better, and more diverse than it was a few years ago, they also reveal some areas of concern that will merit future monitoring.

Interjecting a personal note about the diversity of today's medical students, you might be interested in an incident that took place last month at Howard University medical school, where I am a part-time consultant to the dean's office. Since I had never visited the new university hospital, I joined a group of about twenty entering students for one of their orientation-week tours. Much to my surprise and pleasure, I was asked in all seriousness by several students whether I was a fellow member of their entering class. When this can happen to a fifty-six-year-old white grandfather in a predominantly black medical school, I am convinced that today's students are not only much more diverse but more diplomatic than those of the past.

---

* Arkansas, Case Western Reserve, Chicago-Pritzker, Cincinnati, Colorado, Emory, Harvard, Howard, Iowa, Kentucky, Miami, Stanford, SUNY-Syracuse, and Washington.

Since the theme of the conference is "Recent Trends in Medical Education," most of my comments will deal with the medical student body of 1974–75, as compared with the immediately previous generation of 1970–71. Whereas Joseph Ceithaml focused on the selection for the entering class, I will discuss students in all four classes. In cases where information was not available for the full student body for each of these periods, the closest available data are reported.

QUANTITY

The national medical student body in 1974–75 consisted of 53,554 students, as compared with 40,238 students four years earlier [1] (Table 1). Although the number of medical schools rose from 102 to 114 during those four years, the average size of the student body grew from 394 to 470 students per school. In relation to this growth in class size, one of the concerns being expressed today by medical school faculty and administrators alike is the increasing difficulty of avoiding depersonalization—of ensuring that students are known as individuals by faculty, the dean, and fellow students.

The following recent reactions from student affairs officers at several average-size medical schools illustrate this problem:

● Although our students are competent, interested, and relatively happy, they are definitely desirous of more personal attention than they receive.

● Our first-year faculty complain that unless the students' photographs reach them early, they do not get to know the students well enough to prepare personal evaluations for the dean's office.

TABLE 1. CHARACTERISTICS OF UNITED STATES MEDICAL STUDENTS: QUANTITY

	Base Year 1970–71*	Current Year 1974–75†	Change Number	Percent
Number of students	40,238	53,554	13,316	+33
Number of schools	102	114	12	+12
Average size of student body	394	470	76	+19

Source: W. F. Dubé, "Datagram: U.S. Medical Student Enrollment, 1970–71 Through 1974–75," *Journal of Medical Education* 50, no. 3 (1975).

* Entered 1967, 1968, 1969, and 1970.
† Entered 1971, 1972, 1973, and 1974.

- Because of the Buckley Amendment to the Family Educational Rights and Privacy Act of 1974, which delays publication of the usual lists of students' names and addresses, after five weeks of school our first-year students still do not know each other.
- Have you tried lately to compose over one hundred personal, individualized, internship recommendations per year?

QUALITY

The high academic quality of medical students was maintained and possibly even improved from the 1970–71 to the 1974–75 student body generations (Table 2). In terms of selectivity, for example, the size of the applicant pool for a representative class rose by 66 percent from the early to the mid-1970s, while the number of enrollees increased by only 36 percent over the same period. Whereas the earlier class was selected from 2.35 percent of applicants per enrollee, the later class was chosen from 2.87 percent of candidates per place, for a 22 percent increase in student selectivity as measured by the ratio of applicants to enrollees.[2]

This rise in selectivity is also reflected in the mean undergraduate grade point averages (GPAs) of students in those classes. For example, the latter class had twice as many students with A averages as the earlier class, with the proportion of A students going from 18 percent for 1969 entrants to 36 percent for 1973 entrants.[3]

The Medical College Admission Test (MCAT) scores of those in the 1969 and 1973 entering classes were very high and generally comparable.[4] The latter class scored slightly higher in verbal and quantative ability and fifteen points higher in science, while its mean score on the general information test dropped slightly.

The medical student of 1975 continues to bring with him or her a strong science background. Of those accepted to the 1974 entering class, 85 percent majored in one of the biological or physical sciences or in a premedical program.[5] The only change from the class entering four years earlier was a slight decrease in those reporting a "premedical" major.[6] Contrary to some earlier predictions, humanities majors remained at 6 percent, and social science majors stayed constant at 9 percent of all entrants.

A further indication of the high quality of today's medical students is found in the continued low attrition rates in recent classes.[7, 8] Although the average attrition of all students enrolled rose from 1.03 percent for the 1969–70 student body to 1.41 percent for the

TABLE 2. CHARACTERISTICS OF UNITED STATES MEDICAL STUDENTS: QUALITY

	1970–71 Sopho- mores*	1974–75 Sopho- mores†	Change Number	Change Percent
Applicant Pool [1]				
Number of applicants	24,465	40,506	16,041	+66
Number of enrollees	10,422	14,159‡	3,737	+36
Applicants per enrollee	2.35	2.87	.52	+22
Average Undergraduate	(Percent)	(Percent)		
Grade Point Average [2]				
A (3.6–4.0)	17.9	36.4		+18.5
B (2.6–3.5)	76.6	58.8		−17.8
C (Below 2.6)	5.5	4.8		−0.7
Medical College Admission				
Test Scores of Acceptees [1]				
Verbal ability	562	567	+5	
Quantitative ability	603	609	+6	
General information	569	563	−6	
Science	577	592	+15	
Undergraduate Majors [3,4]	(1971–72 Matriculants, Percent)	(1974–75 Acceptees, Percent)		
Biological and				
physical sciences	75	79	+4	
Premedical	10	6	−4	
Subtotal	(85)	(85)		
Humanities	6	6		
Social sciences	9	9		
Subtotal	(15)	(15)		
Net Attrition Rate [5,6]	(1969–70, Percent)	(1973–74, Percent)		
First year	2.84	2.33		−.51
Intermediate years	.42	1.40		+.98
Final year	.19	.30		+.11
Total	3.45	4.03		+.58
Weighted average	1.03	1.41		+.38

Source: 1) W. F. Dubé, "Datagram: Applicants for the 1973–74 Medical School Entering Class," *Journal of Medical Education* 49, no. 11 (1974); 2) Association of American Medical Colleges, *Medical School Admission Requirements, 1976–77, U.S.A. and Canada*, ed. V. L. Wilson (Washington: Association of American Medical Colleges, 1975); 3) D. G. Johnson, V. C. Smith, and S. L. Tarnoff, "Recruitment and Progress of Minority Medical Entrants, 1970–72: A Cooperative Study by the SNMA and the AAMC," *Journal of Medical Education*, suppl. 50, no. 7 (1975); 4) Association of American Medical Colleges, "AAMC Admissions Action Summary for 1974–75 Entering Class," mimeographed (Washington: Association of American Medical Colleges, 1975); 5) "Medical Education in the United States," *Journal of the American Medical Association* 214, no. 8 (1970); and 6) Anne E. Crowley, ed., "Medical Education in the United States, 1973–74," *Journal of the American Medical Association* suppl. 231 (January 1975).

* Data actually for 1969 entrants.
† Data actually for 1973 entrants.
‡ Higher than number in note 2.

1973–74 body, this is still an extremely low ratio of loss. Even when the average attrition for each class level is totaled to approximate the cumulative dropout rate over four years, approximately 96 percent of today's students can be expected to receive the M.D. degree. This compares with an eventual success rate of only 91 percent when the last AAMC study of attrition was conducted in the 1960s.[9]

Again, these statistics on the "quality" of today's students can be fleshed out by reporting the following typical reactions received recently from deans of students at representative medical schools:

- Our students are brighter and better prepared than ever before.
- Our students are sufficiently scientifically oriented, willing to work hard to improve their understanding, and ready to set extremely high standards for their own performance.
- Our students not only present better admissions credentials than they did in the past, but they also present a much neater appearance —more clothes and less hair!

The only major negative reaction relative to quality was:

- I am seeing more "grim professionals" among our students than ever before. The intense competition for admission has, I believe, caused students while in college to abandon extracurricular experiences or anything that might jeopardize the *A* average. I view this trend with dismay.

DIVERSITY

In many ways the student body of 1974–75 is more diverse than that of four years earlier (Table 3); in other respects, this does not hold true.

Perhaps the major shift has been the increase of women students in our medical schools. Their number rose from 3,878 in 1970–71 to 9,661 in 1974–75.[10] Where they represented 9.6 percent of the student body four short years ago, they constituted 18 percent during the past school year. According to a recent Delphi University survey of medical school deans conducted by the AAMC, it is forecast that the percentage of women will increase to 30 percent by 1985.[11] The continued movement in this direction is confirmed by the fact that in the fall of 1975 approximately 24 percent of the entering class were expected to be women.

A similar substantial increase in diversity has taken place with regard to the racial-ethnic backgrounds of our medical students.

TABLE 3. CHARACTERISTICS OF UNITED STATES MEDICAL STUDENTS: DIVERSITY

	Base Year 1970–71	Current Year 1974–75	Change	
			Number	Percent
Women	3,878 (9.6)*	9,661 (18.0)*	5,783	+149 (+88)
Minority and Foreign Students				
Selected United States minorities				
Black American	1,509	3,355	1,846	+122
American Indian	18	159	141	+783
Mexican American	148	638	490	+331
Puerto Rican—				
Mainland	48	172	124	+258
Subtotal	1,723 (4.3)*	4,324 (8.1)*	2,601	+151
Other United States minorities (mostly American Orientals)	571	1,236	665	+116
Total United States minorities	2,294 (5.7)*	5,560 (10.4)*	3,266	+142
Foreign students	650	819	169	+26
(Non-United States blacks)	(180)	(287)	(107)	(+59)
Total minority and foreign	2,944 (7.4)*	6,379 (11.9)*	3,435	+117

Source: W. F. Dubé, "Datagram: U. S. Medical Student Enrollment, 1970–71 Through 1974–75," *Journal of Medical Education* 50, no. 3 (1975).
* Percent of student body.

Although the number of American minority group students started with a smaller base figure of only 5.7 percent in 1970–71, this grew to 10.4 percent in 1974–75. Accordingly, minority enrollments rose by 142 percent, as compared with a similar 149 percent increase for women. The number of foreign students, although proportionately very low, also went up slightly, from 650 in 1970–71 to 819 in 1974–75. Among these students, incidentally, the number of non-United States blacks rose from 180 to 287.[12]

Another small but significant contributor to diversity is the increased number of transfers to advanced standing. Whereas in 1970–71 fewer than six hundred students transferred to United

States medical schools,[13] almost seven hundred and fifty were admitted to advanced standing in 1973–74, the latest year for which data are available.[14] The latter group included 228 from two-year medical schools; 153 from four-year schools in the United States; 169 from foreign medical schools; and 181 from other degree programs such as osteopathic medicine and dentistry.

Turning to diversity in socioeconomic background, we find less change from 1970–71 to 1974–75 in this area than in sex, race, citizenship, and transfer status (Table 4). Also, in comparison with the United States population at large, there is less diversity in the family heritage of medical students than might have been expected from the recent efforts by many schools to admit more students from nontraditional socioeconomic backgrounds.

Relative to the gross income of their parents, for example, 36 percent of the population in 1974 had family incomes of less than $10,000, whereas only 15 percent of the 1974 medical school entrants came from this income level.[15, 16] Comparable figures at the upper end of the scale were 40 percent with incomes of $15,000 or more, as contrasted with 67 percent of the 1974 entrants.

The relatively high family incomes are consistent with the occupational and educational levels of the fathers of these students. For both the 1970–71 and 1974–75 student bodies, 15 percent and 14 percent, respectively, had fathers who were physicians, and two-thirds were in professional or managerial occupations. Comparable figures in 1970 for employed males aged forty or over were only 1 percent physicians and 26 percent in professional and managerial careers.[17] Conversely, only 19 percent of the 1970–71 medical students had fathers who were skilled, unskilled, or farm workers, as compared with 59 percent of employed males in these occupations. Shifting from the general population to a comparison of the 1974–75 students with their counterparts in 1970–71, there does not appear to have been any significant change in the distribution of their fathers' occupations.[18, 19]

Turning to fathers' education, there does appear to be a slight upgrading for the 1974–75 student body over that in 1970–71. For example, 55 percent of the fathers of the 1974–75 students had at least a college education, compared with 49 percent in 1970–71. Comparable figures for males age forty or over in 1970 show only 11 percent with a college education or better. Similarly, whereas in both periods almost 90 percent of students' fathers had completed

TABLE 4. CHARACTERISTICS OF UNITED STATES MEDICAL STUDENTS:
SOCIOECONOMIC BACKGROUNDS

	Base Year 1970–71 (Percent)	Current Year 1974–75 (Percent)	United States Population, 1974 (Percent)
Gross Income of Parents [1]			
Less than $5,000		5	13
$5,000–$9,999		10	23
$10,000–$14,999		18	24
$15,000–$19,999		14	} 40
$20,000 or more		53	

Employed Males, Age 40+, 1970

	Base Year	Current Year	United States Population
Father's Occupation [1,2]			
Physician	15	14	1
Other health worker	5	5	1
Other professional and technical	28	29	11
Owner, manager, proprietor	20	23	14
Clerical and sales	12	10	14
Skilled worker	10	10	22
Unskilled worker	6	6	31
Farmer, farm worker	3	4	6

					United States Males, Age 40+, 1970	
Father's Education [1,2]	(Percent)	(Cumulative percent)	(Percent)	(Cumulative percent)	(Percent)	(Cumulative percent)
Graduate or professional	35	35	38	38	5	5
Completed college	14	49	17	55	6	11
Some college (or technical school)	20	69	18	73	9	20
Completed high school	17	86	15	88	23	43
Some high school	6	92	5	93	19	62
Eighth grade or less	8	100	7	100	38	100

Source: 1) J. A. Lambdin, "Survey of How Medical Students Finance Their Education 1974–75," mimeographed (Washington: Association of American Medical Colleges, 1975); 2) U.S. Department of Health, Education, and Welfare, *How Medical Students Finance Their Education,* DHEW Publication No. 75–13 (Washington: Department of Health, Education, and Welfare, 1974).

at least a high school education, only 43 percent of the males age forty or above had reached this educational level in 1970.[20, 21]

Although not shown in the tables, comparable figures for the mothers of medical students reveal that they also are increasingly a highly educated group. For example, whereas 50 percent of students' mothers in 1970–71 had at least some college, according to the preliminary findings this proportion rose to 57 percent in 1974–75.[22, 23]

A much greater change has taken place in the marital status of medical students than in their family backgrounds (Table 5). According to preliminary data, only 38 percent of all 1974–75 students were married, a sizeable drop from the 47 percent of the 1970–71 group. The contrast is particularly striking for seniors, with the proportion dipping from 65 percent in 1970–71 to 52 percent in 1974–75.[24, 25] According to an informal poll of student affairs officers, these changes in marital status are consistent with both an increased divorce rate and a trend for today's young people to live together for a period instead of being officially married.

To supplement the statistics on diversity, I would like once again to report a few recent comments from medical school officials:

- Our students today represent great diversity. For example, approximately half of our last entering class are either minority or female.
- Our student body includes not only more women and minority group members, but also such widely diverse individuals as Catholic nuns and professional football players. Their presence is chang-

TABLE 5. CHARACTERISTICS OF MEDICAL STUDENTS:
MARITAL STATUS

	Base Year 1970–71	Current Year 1974–75	Percent Change
Percent Married [1]			
First year	35	25	−10
Second year	41	40 }	−6 }
Third year	51		
Final year	65	52	−13
All classes	47	38	−9

Source: 1) J. A. Lambdin, "Survey of How Medical Students Finance Their Education 1974–75," mimeographed (Washington: Association of American Medical Colleges, 1975); 2) U.S. Department of Health, Education, and Welfare, *How Medical Students Finance Their Education,* DHEW Publication No. 75–13 (Washington: Department of Health, Education, and Welfare, 1974).

ing the attitudes of our faculty and staff about students with unusual
backgrounds.

- Although our student body is currently very diverse, I'm concerned
  that further restrictions in financial aid will cause us to revert to
  medical school classes coming almost entirely from affluent professional families.
- Our student body in 1975 is far more diverse than it was in the
  past. This diversity extends to age, sex, race, economic level, social
  background, cultural values, educational background, and career
  goals.

ATTITUDES AND VALUES

As indicated in the last quotation, there is so much diversity in
student attitudes and values it is difficult to make any generalizations that apply to *the* medical student of 1975.

One of our most senior student affairs officers reported to me
recently, for example, that his current students ranged all the way
from:

- The *traditional standard breed* who will fall easily into a conservative professional role; to
- The *solid production types* who are eagerly awaiting the chance to
  produce technically competent services and to enjoy the financial
  and other rewards derived therefrom; to
- The *potential innovators* who have the capacity to become excited
  and involved if they receive a strong external stimulus at the right
  time; to
- The *self-propelling adventurers* who at least temporarily have escaped from the materialistic values of our society and are sincerely
  seeking personal and professional satisfaction through altruistic involvement in the health care system.

My own guess is that nationally we are seeing an increase in the
more conservative, traditional, and production types, and a slight
decrease in the potential innovators and adventurers. All four types
are needed in the health care system, however, and no value judg-
ments are intended either by me or by our "senior" official.

In spite of the variability illustrated among these medical students
I believe at least three major generalizations can be drawn about
how today's students differ from those of the recent past with regard
to their attitudes and values: 1) more outspoken concern about
their own personal welfare; 2) the use of more constructive tactics

for expressing these concerns; and 3) more active interest in the provision of primary care to underserved areas.

Elaborating on the first generalization, it is apparent that students are more willing to express concern not only about their own personal growth and development, but about preserving human dignity and privacy. They are more open in expressing their feelings to the faculty relative to both the quality of teaching and to the methods of presentation. Male, female, and minority students have joined together at some schools, for example, to formally petition male faculty members to refrain from the use of sexist or racist humor in their lectures.

Other examples may be found in: 1) the strong student support of the Buckley Amendment to protect the privacy of their own records; and 2) the new student advocacy system of the American Medical Student Association (AMSA)—formerly the Student American Medical Association (SAMA)—which seeks to help protect student rights at the institutional level.[26]

Medical students and their spouses are also insisting on more time for rest and recreation, rather than devoting all of their waking hours to the study of medicine. As one dean of students reported to me recently:

- More of our students are now willing to admit that medicine is not the be-all and end-all of their existence.

This growing insistence on personal and professional development is consistent with the current societal emphasis on human liberation and consciousness raising. These values are also reinforced by having larger numbers of women and minorities in the student body, as well as by recent federal legislation in the areas of affirmative action and the protection of privacy.

The second major generalization about today's medical students is that most of them are now using tactics of cooperation and communication rather than those of confrontation and demonstration that were so common in the 1960s and early 1970s during the days of Vietnam, Cambodia, and Kent State.[27] Representative quotes on this theme from my student affairs colleagues include the following:

- Courtesy is returning, while frankness remains. That is, our students still feel free to express discontent, but they do so less angrily. Our students are returning to a posture that resembles that of the early 1960s. While they maintain their social concern, and demonstrate this by working in free clinics, by tutoring, and by undertaking masters' programs in various public health areas, they're not nearly as strident or belligerent in expressing their concerns.

- Our school has seen a major shift in student attitudes. Not only have the students changed with the end of the Vietnam War, but the medical school faculty and administration may have reduced the need for overactivism by including students in planning and decision making.

Finally, the third major generalization about student values is their increasing interest in the fields of primary care and in the provision of such care to patients in underserved areas.

Preliminary data from the 1974–75 AAMC survey of "How Medical Students Finance their Education" [28] indicate, for example, that over 90 percent of today's students are planning on careers in patient care, rather than in research, teaching, or administration. Similarly, over 50 percent of those with specialty plans are aiming for primary care, broadly defined, that is, family medicine, general internal medicine, general pediatrics, and obstetrics and gynecology. Approximately 50 percent of the students also report an interest in working in a medically underserved area, with rural locations being somewhat preferred over urban areas.

A few quotes from recent communications from colleagues may serve to illustrate these career choice trends:

- We have more students planning careers in family medicine—but as general internists and general pediatricians, rather than as general family physicians.
- Students at our school are showing a greatly increased interest in primary care. They are more interested in patients than in diseases and have more concern regarding community health.
- At our school there is a growing concern on the part of all students regarding the health care delivery system, its organization, the manpower required, and the question of payment.

Why are today's students showing these shifts in career goals and interests? I believe it is due in part to the admissions process, which has increasingly tried to select students who are most apt to meet society's perceived needs for more primary care and for better geographical distribution of health services. Both students and admissions committees are also undoubtedly affected by existing governmental and private programs, such as the National Health Service Corps, federal and state loan forgiveness for practice in underserved areas, and the $10 million Robert Wood Johnson Student Aid

Program for students who are female, from rural areas, and/or from a minority group.[29]

Furthermore, they are aware of the "handwriting on the wall," which indicates potentially drastic changes in future programs of student aid as well as in career opportunities. As described by one medical school colleague:

- The bills in Congress that would further control the type and geographic location of practice, although not yet law, are having a marked effect on what students are thinking about career choices.

STUDENT ORGANIZATIONS

Additional evidence of the three generalizations cited earlier about recent changes in student attitudes and values can be found in a comparison of the activities of the major national medical student organizations in 1970–71 and in 1974–75.

Relative to student concerns about their own welfare, for example, the official report of the 1974 annual meeting of the SAMA starts with the following paragraph:

If you're a medical student, you can expect SAMA to be going to bat for you this year. In an unprecedented switch in priorities, the 1974 SAMA House of Delegates, meeting in Dallas, demanded that the national organization take positive steps to come to the aid of medical students at the local level.[30]

The report goes on to indicate that this change in emphasis is best illustrated by two resolutions passed by its House of Delegates, which call for protection of medical students' rights. These resolutions dealt with violations of the confidentiality of students' records, and the excessive amounts of time students are expected to spend doing "scut work." The latter resolution, incidentally, urged that schools provide for students to have at least five uninterrupted hours of sleep out of every twenty-four. To this observer, whose son is now a fourth-year medical student, that does not appear to be too unreasonable a request.

Similarly, a recent publication of the Student National Medical Association (SNMA), the *Student Rights Handbook,* informs minority students, in particular, of their legal rights on such matters as due process, judicial review of administrative proceedings, right to counsel, and the confidentiality of student records.[31] The handbook also illustrates the general trend toward working within the system.

This shift in emphasis is further evidenced by comparing the SAMA resolutions of 1970 with those of 1975. In 1970, seventy-five resolutions were introduced, the last two of which are of particular relevance to this presentation.[32] One called for vigorous action on individual college campuses in opposition to the Indo-Chinese war, with emphasis to be placed on activities during the two weeks prior to the 1970 fall congressional elections so that students could campaign for peace candidates and oppose supporters of the war. The other resolution passed by the House of Delegates provided for the SAMA convention to adjourn early to allow a large number of the members to attend the May 1970 Washington Peace March; it resolved that the association should give open support to the march by announcing to the media its intention to participate as an easily identifiable group carrying a SAMA banner.

By contrast, the 1975 SAMA convention considered only thirty-three resolutions,* most of which dealt with procedural matters such as changing its name, supporting house staff strikes, and trying to open to the public the AMA's Liaison Committee on Medical Education accreditation records, reports, and deliberations.[33]

The reports of its 1975 annual meeting also headlined the fact that it had elected its first national woman president, Laurel Coppa, a thirty-three year-old, third-year student at Case-Western Reserve. It is noteworthy in this International Women's Year that the SNMA likewise installed its first woman president, Virginia Davis, a third-year student at Howard University.

These student leaders and their constituents give evidence of the previously cited student interest in primary care. Ms. Coppa, for example, says that one of her major goals for the coming year is "to see AMSA develop model primary-care curricula and to work with local students to get medical schools to adopt such programs." She also hopes "to work toward developing ethics seminars and workshops for medical students that would cover such problems as physician maldistribution. . . ."[34]

Related actions in 1975 by both AMSA and SNMA included continued support for national efforts to promote the enrollment of minority students in schools of the health professions.[35, 36]

SUMMARY AND CONCLUSION

I would characterize medical students in 1975 as being not only greater in quantity, but better in academic quality, more evenly

---

* The national headquarters of AMSA, 5 September 1975: personal communication.

distributed by sex, and much more diverse in racial background than their counterparts of even four short years ago.

The shift in the socioeconomic backgrounds of the students has not been great, however, and, if anything, we may find an even larger proportion of students from wealthy backgrounds in the future unless adjustments are made in the financial aid situation.

Student attitudes and values appear to be shifting in the directions of: 1) more explicit concern about their own welfare; 2) more constructive tactics for expressing these concerns; and 3) greater interest in primary medical care.

Overall, today's students are still a very choice group of individuals, and the future of medicine should be excellent if their expected contributions are fulfilled.

In the words of my colleagues in student affairs:

- As a group, today's medical students are very stimulating people, clearly selected from near the top of their peers in terms of ability, personality, and character.
- Our students are respectful, pleasant to work with, helpful to others, and truly desirous of becoming the finest M.D.'s possible. They are, in fact, a delight to be associated with.

Lest my colleagues and I be accused of being too Pollyanna-ish, however, I must report in closing that several of them expressed heightened concern that today's students are retaining many of the "cutthroat competition" characteristics they needed to get into medical school. For this reason they recommend that in the future even more attention should be focused on the assessment and nourishment of positive personal qualities. As one associate dean put it:

- I believe that faculties of medical schools should define in greater depth and detail the noncognitive requirements for receipt of the M.D. degree. I'm impressed, as a result of student problems faced during 1974–75, that this is probably of even more importance than are the definition and enforcement of academic standards.

Along these same lines, other respondents emphasized the need to move ahead vigorously with such national activities as the AAMC Simulated Admissions Exercise [37] and the noncognitive portion of the new Medical College Admissions Assessment Program,[38] which will soon be replacing the MCAT.

In conclusion, therefore, I believe that while the medical student in 1975 is very much alive and well, we must continue to improve our admissions, student affairs, financial aid, and career counseling programs if we want to assure that the medical student of the 1980s will be of equally high quality. Even though this assurance will require a considerable investment of time, effort, and money, it will be more than justified if one accepts my opening thesis that the most important single ingredient in determining the success of medical education is the caliber of the individual student.

Notes

1. W. F. Dubé, "Datagram: U.S. Medical Student Enrollment, 1970–71 Through 1974–75," *Journal of Medical Education,* 50, no. 3 (1975): 303–06.

2. ———, "Datagram: Applicants for the 1973–74 Medical School Entering Class," *Journal of Medical Education,* 49, no. 11 (1974): 1070–72.

3. Association of American Medical Colleges, *Medical School Admission Requirements, 1976–77, U.S.A. and Canada,* ed. V. L. Wilson (Washington: Association of American Medical Colleges, 1975).

4. Dubé, "1973–74 Medical School Entering Class" (see note 2).

5. Association of American Medical Colleges, "AAMC Admissions Action Summary for 1974–75 Entering Class," mimeographed (Washington: Association of American Medical Colleges, 1975).

6. D. G. Johnson, V. C. Smith, and S. L. Tarnoff, "Recruitment and Progress of Minority Medical School Entrants, 1970–1972," *Journal of Medical Education,* suppl. 50, no. 7 (1975): 713–55.

7. "Medical Education in the United States, 1969–70," *Journal of the American Medical Association* 214, no. 8 (1970): 1483–1581.

8. Anne E. Crowley, ed., "Medical Education in the United States, 1973–1974," *Journal of the American Medical Association,* suppl. 231 (January 1975): 1–139.

9. D. G. Johnson and E. B. Hutchins, "Doctor or Dropout? A Study of Medical Student Attrition," *Journal of Medical Education,* 49, no. 12 (1966): 1099–1269.

10. Dubé, "Enrollment 1970–71 Through 1974–75" (see note 1).

11. J. A. Keyes, M. P. Wilson, and J. Becker, "The Future of Medical Education: Forecast of the Council of Deans," *Journal of Medical Education,* 50, no. 4 (1975): 319–27.

12. Dubé, "Enrollment 1970–71 Through 1974–75" (see note 1).

13. "Medical Education, 1969–70" (see note 7).

14. Crowley, ed., "Medical Education, 1973–1974" (see note 8).

15. J. A. Lambdin, "Survey of How Medical Students Finance Their Education, 1974–75," mimeographed (Washington: Association of American Medical Colleges, 1975).

16. U.S. Bureau of the Census, "Money Income and Poverty Status of Families and Persons in the United States: 1974," in *Current Population Reports,* Series P-60, No. 99 (Washington: U.S. Government Printing Office, 1974).

17. U.S. Department of Health, Education, and Welfare, *How Medical Students Finance Their Education,* DHEW Publication No. 75–13 (Washington: Department of Health, Education, and Welfare, 1974).

18. Lambdin, "How Medical Students Finance Education" (see note 15).
19. Department of Health, Education, and Welfare, *How Students Finance Education* (see note 17).
20. Lambdin, "How Medical Students Finance Education" (see note 15).
21. Department of Health, Education, and Welfare, *How Students Finance Education* (see note 17).
22. Lambdin, "How Medical Students Finance Education" (see note 15).
23. Department of Health, Education, and Welfare, *How Students Finance Education* (see note 17).
24. Lambdin, "How Medical Students Finance Education" (see note 15).
25. Department of Health, Education, and Welfare, *How Students Finance Education* (see note 17).
26. C. Rice, "SAMA in 1974," *New Physician* 23 (1974): 32–34.
27. D. G. Johnson, "Medical Student Admission, Attrition, and Activism," *New Physician* 17 (1968): 23–28.
28. Lambdin, "How Medical Students Finance Education" (see note 15).
29. Association of American Medical Colleges, *Admission Requirements, 1976–77, U.S.A. and Canada* (see note 3).
30. Rice, "SAMA in 1974" (see note 26).
31. J. A. Burt, *Preliminary Student Rights Handbook* (Washington: Student National Medical Association, 1972).
32. "Resolutions of the 1970 SAMA House of Delegates," *New Physician* 19 (1970): 582–90.
33. C. Rice, "SAMA Delegates Change Name, Elect First Woman President," *New Physician* 24 (1975): 14–15.
34. ———, "Woman Wins Top AMSA Post," Ibid.: 16.
35. Ibid.
36. W. H. Hall and Y. Davis, "The SNMA 11th Annual Medical Education Conference March 27–30, 1975," mimeographed, Report to the HEW Office of Health Resources Opportunity by the Student National Medical Association, Washington, 1975, mimeographed (Washington: Student National Medical Association, 1975).
37. A. G. D'Costa, et al., *Simulated Admissions Exercise: An Approach to the Appraisal of Nontraditional Applicants to Medical Schools* (Washington: Association of American Medical Colleges, 1975).
38. Association of American Medical Colleges, *Admission Requirements, 1976–77* (see note 3).

ॐ

DISCUSSION

The discussion opened with a consideration of attrition rates. Studies made by Johnson in the early 1960s suggested a 7 percent attrition rate as ideal. Today, with the overall rate at 1.41 percent, the pendulum is considered to have swung too far, in part at least because of capitation pressures. Students themselves complain that too many of their poorly qualified peers are allowed to graduate.

A new phenomenon was reported: a growing number of students not in academic difficulty are "running out of steam" at the end of their first year of medical school, or the beginning of their second; they are psychologically tired and wish to take a year off from their studies. This is attributable to the intense pressure and competition of the premedical years, a state of affairs that continues during the first year of medical school. These students are now asking themselves, "Do I really want to be a doctor?" Unfortunately there appears to be no way at present to screen out these students in the admissions process, or to lessen the battlefield-like atmosphere of the premedical period.

A similar problem exists among older students with advanced placement in both the sciences and the humanities. Because they are thrown into the clinical phase of their medical studies at an early stage, many are experiencing difficulties in the area of noncognitive skills. Giving their first physical examination, for example, can be a traumatic experience.

On the subject of minority representation, it was emphasized that women should not be included in this category. A subtle form of discrimination against women does, of course, exist. A Johns Hopkins University study showed that the perseverance rate for eventual admittance on the part of rejected male applicants is higher than that for women. One reason for this is that women receive less encouragement from their advisors than do their male counterparts.

It was noted that although the AAMC target rate for ethnic minority enrollment in medical school for 1975 was 12 percent, minority students actually comprise only 8 percent of the 1975–76 class.

More diversity now exists in the economic backgrounds of ethnic minority students, with an increasing number coming from the middle class. This is the result of two factors: pressure from middle-class blacks, who believe their children who are qualified for admission to medical school are being passed over in favor of economically disadvantaged minority students; and increasingly stringent financial conditions imposed by the federal government, in the form of lower capitation grants and reductions in funds for student loans. (One participant remarked that at her school, some students were graduating with debts of $20,000.) These financial conditions are seen as an urgent problem. Without economic assistance, medical schools are in danger of returning to all-white, upper-middle-class student bodies. The solution appears to lie with the Congress.

A New Paradigm for Medical Education

LAWRENCE L. WEED

In a conference on "Trends in Medical Education" one could discuss one's views as to what is happening and what is likely to happen, given our present premises and tools, or one could discuss what could happen if our premises and tools were changed. I shall do the latter.

First, why new tools and premises? It is our belief that serious inadequacies have appeared in the present medical care system, and that some of our present educational premises and tools are at least partly responsible.

The paper that follows is divided into four sections. The first deals with the structure of the present medical care and educational systems; certain flaws in the structure will be reviewed. The second presents two tools—the manual, problem-oriented medical record (POMR) and the computerized POMR—to deal with these flaws; the philosophical basis for shifting to such tools will be presented. The third presents new premises on which medical education should be based, which derive logically from the issues discussed in the first two sections. The fourth consists of a discussion of how the new tools and new premises combine to allow practical implementation of a curriculum for medicine.

INADEQUACIES LEAD TO NEW TOOLS AND NEW PREMISES

The inadequacies are:

1. Lack of coordination of information among providers;
2. Failure of the record to unambiguously and consistently preserve the logic of actions, as well as evidence of the actions themselves;
3. Unrealistic use of and dependence on human memory; and

4. Lack of meaningful feedback loops on everyday medical action—the system is blind.

First a framework is needed in which to think about these inadequacies. In medical care, like any other organized endeavor, there should be:

- A system or a structure with rules;
- Audit of performance within the rules and correction of the deficiencies; and
- Audit of the system itself by examining outcomes, and a change in the system when necessary.

What is our present medical system and how did it develop? Let us go back to the days of a single patient and a single physician in a small town, for example. In this system the doctor often recorded little, but, because he lived near the patient, by daily exposure he knew much about his or her social, psychiatric, and medical history. Furthermore, there was much less precise scientific knowledge and fewer techniques, and few if any specialists interacted with their patients.

Then, as the body of knowledge grew and doctors continued to believe they should learn it, memorize it, and pass examinations, they started to specialize. They also legitimately specialized to develop new surgical techniques and new technologies such as radiology. So now we have a single patient relating to several physicians (Figure 1).

Some of these physicians, such as the radiologist, dealt with the patient mainly in a technical sense and did not presume to provide total care. As further advances came, these physicians were supported by a series of specialists, hidden as far as the patient was concerned—pathologists, biochemists, and so forth. Then each field developed ancillary medical personnel, and a single patient was surrounded by a large number of people. It was inevitable that a problem of coordination of medical information would develop. The right hand did now know what the left hand was doing. The cardiologist prescribing one drug was unaware that his drug was being antagonized by another given by the psychiatrist; indeed he may not have known his patient was going to a psychiatrist. Even if he had, however, because of the sheer mass of detail in modern medicine, it is unlikely that either physician would have been aware that the two drugs antagonized one another.

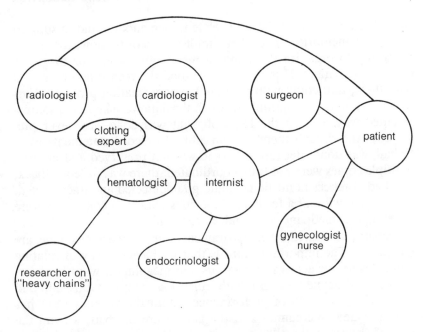

Figure 1. Relationship of a Patient to Several Physicians.

To make matters worse, a given patient may not see a given doctor, nurse, or medical worker over a long period of time, even within a given area of specialization, due to the increased mobility of both medical personnel and patients. The resulting provincialism, in time as well as in space, has led, to use le Corbusier's phrase, to "a spectacle of fragments of intention." In such a situation, cost-benefit analysis applied to one of the fragments can be very misleading. One hasty, episodic bit of care to save a few minutes and dollars in a clinic, only to generate costs of hundreds of dollars for care in an expensive hospital months later, cannot show up in the cost-benefit analysis of the clinic alone. Emergency rooms in hospitals are rarely thought of as part of the feedback loop and a source of valuable end-stage information that should be used to modify behavior at other points in the loop. They rarely try to control the inflow by dealing with basic causes. They just expand and seek more money. Medical faculties and specialties position themselves at various disconnected points in these potential cycles and elaborate on their expertise to handle the problem at hand.

In an effort to solve the coordination problem, medical personnel started to keep records, both to relate to one another and to support their own memories. They kept multiple records, however, never bothering to organize them into a meaningful whole or to give a copy to the patient. If patients understood the record and carried it with them, that could help to solve the coordination problem. Furthermore, in the old multiple records, the data were kept in a source-oriented way, so that the logic of what was done was never preserved, even though there was an effort to record statements as to "what" was done. Because the logic was not preserved and because multiple copies were not fully coordinated, there was little feedback, and bad practices in medicine could go undetected and uncorrected. Any system without a feedback loop runs wild, and conditions were so set up that medicine could indeed run wild.

Debates on benefits versus drawbacks in modern medicine are increasing. The important point is that we have no way of relating outcomes to our actions in rigorous and meaningful ways because: 1) no well-defined system with rules has been established; and 2) no rigorous audit of performance within the system's rules has been pursued. We cannot sort the good from the bad; we run the risk of trying to do all, and going bankrupt and hurting people unreasonably. Or we can stop it all irrationally, and throw the baby out with the bathwater.

If we add to our diagram another circle, and fill it full of educators, researchers, and scholars of all types, we have what has developed into the present medical educational system (Figure 2).

Educators took the body of medical knowledge and tried with various teaching techniques, in a modern setting of objectives and examinations, to put that knowledge into the heads of potential physicians, nurses, and other medical personnel. In many instances they assumed it would be used safely in the care of the patient. Medical faculties specialized to an enormous degree to make sure as much information as possible was covered, even though the single student mind could easily suffer from a sensory overload under such circumstances. We fell into the trap of thinking that giving an examination for knowledge at one point in time would ensure performance at that time and for years to come. Even worse, we believed that such transmission of a core of knowledge was necessary and fundamental to good performance.

This then is the system that has evolved: it lacks coordination among its various parts; lacks preservation of the logic of each

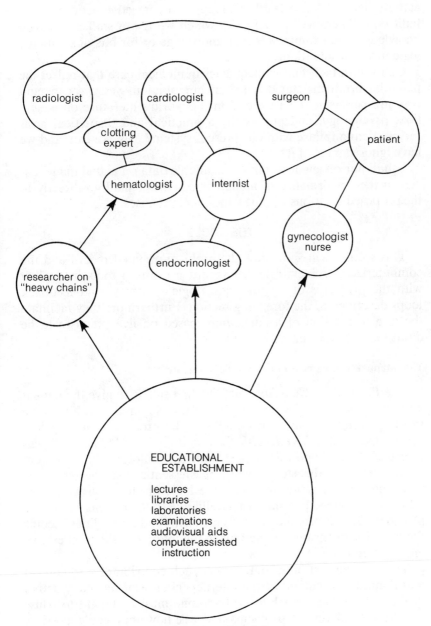

Figure 2. The Present Medical Educational System.

activity; lacks reliable feedback loops and corrective action; and is built on a "memory" principle in which we try to stuff heads with knowledge and examine for that knowledge or for bits of simulated logic in unreal situations.

Can we, in fact, find inadequacies in medical care that reflect the potential problems stated here? In our opinion, yes, we can, and they are pervasive. Can we find in the world's literature on education, psychology, and philosophy a practical and theoretical basis for predicting failure with our present system? Yes, we can, and we have ignored most of it.

I shall not review in detail the available data on actual inadequacies in the performance in modern medicine; I shall go directly to the proposed solutions with new tools and premises.

THE TOOLS

This section will show how the problem-oriented record and the computerized problem-oriented record are useful tools in dealing with the problems of coordination, logic, memory, and feedback loops described in the foregoing section. Furthermore they facilitate the implementation of a curriculum based on five premises to be discussed later (see pages 79–88).

The Manual Problem-Oriented Medical Record

The Problem of Coordination. The first step is to give the patient a copy of his record, which he should always have with him when in the presence of any provider. Begin the process of helping him use it: the book, *Your Health Care and How to Manage It,*[1] was prepared to facilitate this step at both the philosophical and technical levels. For this step to work, it is essential that the record be in a standard form that preserves the logic of all the providers, so all the interconnecting links are intelligible to the patient and to the providers. In this way the patient's problems and capabilities become the basis for integrating all actions in the interest of the total care of an individual.

The problem list immediately puts each contributor into context and reminds the patient of the interdependence of his many activities, problems, and capabilities. Everyone must be taught to pause and look at his list of problems and ask how they could possibly relate to one another in meaningful ways. No plans for solving one problem should be finalized without some thought about its implications for the management of the others. It is at this point that patients and providers must consciously set priorities. A patient has health problems in the first place because of contradictory forces working within his mind and body; the medical profession, through specialization, may add further contradictory forces and make him worse unless they have tools to prevent this from happening.

The Logic Problem. The titled plans and progress notes preserve the logic of each provider so others can see it. The notes must be randomly audited for reliability in representing the patient's true situation, as well as for their intrinsic logic and efficiency of thought and action in the pursuit of the single problem. When the system is first used it is suddenly revealed that goals have not been set; progress notes do not relate to original plans; random thoughts are left dangling; excessive laboratory work is performed; unnecessary risks are taken; and patients are confused about the process in which their cooperation is necessary for the best results. At this point one should not become angry with the POMR. Do not destroy the messenger because you do not like the message; thank the messenger and proceed to deal with the problems revealed.

In the initial plan the physicians, nurse, and patient are to be the architects; in the titled progress notes they and all other medical personnel become the contractors. The teacher is the auditor of the process. All should learn from the process, as human and biological situations unfold.

The Memory Problem. If each provider sees the same POMR, and if the patient has a copy, there is far less chance that a given problem will be dealt with out of context or that others will be overlooked. A provider should not take pride in how much he remembers about a patient; he should be continually aware that his mind alone cannot recall all he should know at each contact in order to give the best possible care. Because one banker may remember figures better than another does not justify giving up the use of bookkeeping systems in banking. Furthermore, the POMR facilitates the development of the physician's capacity to formulate and solve problems, using books, journals, and consultants as necessary. It allows us to audit the logical application of knowledge to patients' needs without determining whether the physician "knew" the knowledge, as opposed to merely developing the habit and skills to use references and consultants effectively (Figure 3).

Feedback Loops. We stated at the outset that we should have: 1) a system with rules; 2) audit of performance within the system

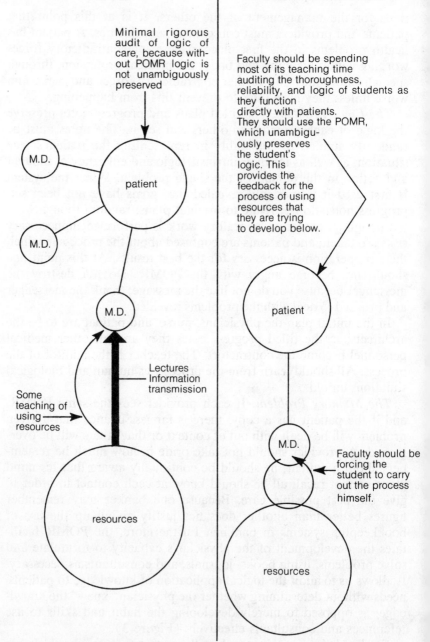

THE OLD   THE NEW WITH THE POMR

Minimal rigorous audit of logic of care, because without POMR logic is not unambiguously preserved

M.D.

patient

M.D.

M.D.

Some teaching of using resources

Lectures
Information
transmission

resources

Faculty should be spending most of its teaching time auditing the thoroughness, reliability, and logic of students as they function directly with patients. They should use the POMR, which unambiguously preserves the student's logic. This provides the feedback for the process of using resources that they are trying to develop below.

patient

M.D.

Faculty should be forcing the student to carry out the process himself.

resources

Figure 3. The Old and the New Systems with the POMR.

and corrective action; and 3) audit of the system itself with outcomes, and correct it when necessary. The system is made up of leads, resources, personnel, messages, and communication tools. The POMR represents the structure and the rules for communicating over time; it is the basis for the feedback loop. Outcomes should not be interpreted until, in terms of the rules, performance is good. Otherwise the system may be prematurely criticized and altered. Continuously operating feedback loops with a well-defined system form the basis for reaching goals. The POMR is the principal tool within the system. While the tool itself guarantees nothing, without it, consequences cannot be related to means and the loop is broken.

The Computerized Problem-Oriented Medical Record

The role of the computerized POMR can be facilitated if we relate to our first three diagrams and extend them. The changes are major and the implications are far-reaching (Figure 4).

All administrative and medical personnel go from papers and pens, dictaphones and typewriters, messages and telephones to a television-like, touch-sensitive screen (a computer terminal) from which they make choices.

A computer serves the terminal holding the TV-like screen by providing the displays from which the choices are made. All the resources from which medical knowledge can arise must be utilized to build the displays in the computer. All the knowledge must be organized into displays from which choices can be made in logical sequence. Each logical sequence forms a structure that gives orders to the content it holds, and each in turn is the content of the larger structure, the POMR. After data on patients accumulate in the computer in a highly organized manner, such data properly analyzed will become one of the principal sources of outcome data with which we correct the system itself. This can be done only after performance has been brought to a redefined level of thoroughness and reliability when dealing with the patient, using the appropriate tools, and when the context of the data is large enough to be meaningful to a whole individual and not just to one of his organs on a specialty service.

The loop is complete. The role of human memory has been changed—at no point is it directly in the loop, and no longer is the system memory-dependent. The boundaries among administration, patient, all medical personnel, and specialty divisions fall away. The

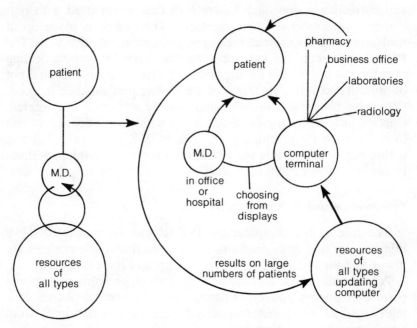

Figure 4. The Role of the Computerized POMR.

autonomy * of separate departments in the medical care system has been broken. The structure of the medical and computer software is based on organizing and pursuing the patient's problems; such a structure cuts across and obliterates the old boundaries that evolved among providers. Furthermore, the boundaries among coordination, memory, logic, and feedback also fall away: they merge into one another. To have perfect coordination and reliable feedback control, factual recall must be removed from the loop, and that can only be done by establishing logical connections among all elements in the computer system. New elements can be entered, but not at random; their place in the structure is determined by the logic by which the structure is constructed.

The overall integrity of the logical structure is forced by a single characteristic of the system, that is, you can proceed only one step at a time by choosing one display at a time. The vast amount of medical knowledge that has been fed into the computer is available

---

* This is one of the main roots of our problem with overutilization, overprofessionalization, and poor distribution and application of resources.

in no other way.* And no display from which you begin, and by which you must proceed, can be independent of the structure of the POMR.

Let us proceed through the system, step by step, and explore some of the requirements and some of the implications that flow from the foregoing discussion.[2]

As a user sits down at a terminal he touches that portion of the screen that states the category of user appropriate to him. A list of users comes up and he selects his name and proceeds to make choices that form his code, thus entering the system. He is then confronted with a list of patients appropriate to him, and, after choosing one, arrives at a basic display from which he picks out that portion of the POMR he wants to use—for example, the data base, the problem list, the initial plans, or the progress notes. One side of the screen is for adding to the record, and the other for retrieving from the record.

If the user elects to add a progress note, for example, he touches "progress note" on the display and immediately the patient's problem list appears. He must choose a problem—his logic has been captured. Then appears the display, asking him the type of information he wants to add with respect to that problem, or the type of order he would like to make, that is, does he want symptomatic information or diagnostic steps. His logic is further delineated and determined before the computer memory yields specific details from which he can select. The choices he makes are either stored in the patient's record alone, or else they are stored and lead to an order at a nurse's station, to a pharmacy, to a radiology department, or to a financial statement in a business office.

The user need not carry in his memory all the options appropriate to his problem or task, but the price he must pay to have at his fingertips such depth of information (literally thousands of displays and hundreds of thousands of choices) is to reveal where he is in his thinking, to relate directly and precisely to the logic pathways built into the computer, and to have the computerized POMR be the complete and sole record of the individual's health. The displays, with their multiple choices, can only come to him one at a time, and each is tightly coupled to the logic of the previous selection. It is true

---

* One step can represent the synthesis and application of a great deal of medical knowledge, just as one mathematical formula can represent an extensive understanding of mathematics. For this reason the users' pathways can be efficient, rather than annoying and cumbersome. At the same time, the precise and full documentation for each action can be ascertained.

that a choice from a display may lead only to information and not to action, or to a theoretical explanation or discussion of criteria, but even that comes one step at a time and always returns the user to where he was in the POMR.

Contrast this procedure with a library, a lecture, a pharmacy, or a conference, in which there are almost an infinite number of opportunities to absorb information without any obligation to couple it to previous logic or future action. The librarian or journal editor is unable to determine or affect the information that has been extracted, how or whether it is stored or used, and whether it is remembered, forgotten, misinterpreted, or distorted over time. As a result, the editor may only be interested in how many journals have been distributed. And when a patient is subjected to medical action of any type it is not unambiguously known what the sources of the information were or what logic led to the actions upon him. The noncomputerized systems of the library and present patient care activities are uncoupled.

Returning to the computerized POMR, not only is a single user tightly coupled to all parts of the system and to sharply defined logic pathways, but multiple users at multiple terminals are coupled to the same system, and therefore to one another. Lewis Mumford has stated that one of the great powers of the clock in the early days of technology was that it could synchronize the actions of man; a great power of the computer is that it can coordinate the actions of man and thereby widen our perception of the consequences of what we do.

At first these ideas seem dehumanizing, the very antithesis of freedom and art and individualism. Yet consider the symphony. How many of us think of it as dehumanizing or the antithesis of art, even though it requires one hundred people playing at the same time to come under the direction of a single individual, and to be guided by a score composed by yet another. We do not think of the musicians as slaves to a dead man's wishes, whose fulfillment is being demanded by some tyrant. Rather we focus on the result and magnificence of the creation. In using the computerized POMR the requirements are not nearly as demanding as those for a member of an orchestra. Physicians and patients do not proceed through identical pathways, simultaneously, the way members of the symphony must play together.

The medical experts have created logically arranged, medical care possibilities in the displays, and the medical personnel use only those that fit the patient's symptoms or problems. There are options at each step, and the final care for any one person emerges slowly: the patient's uniqueness extracts correct choices at each step from the infinitude of possible pathways offered by the computer. At the end of the process, that unique pattern is clear and complete—but no one could have predicted that at the outset.

The logical sequencing of the displays has its origin in the basic structure of the POMR—each level of content in a given structure becomes the structure of the next level of content. For example, the physical examination is content for the data-base structure, the heart examination is content for the physical examination structure, and the auscultation is content for the heart examination structure.

It is this process of delineating content in structures and structures within content that increases the amount of information in a precise and controlled manner. As successive steps are taken, each medical record that emerges is different from every other, emphasizing the uniqueness of individuals. Paradoxically, the very tool we feared would be dehumanizing enables the relentless pursuit of the pathways that establish both the large and subtle differences in individual requirements. One rapidly goes beyond the capacity of the human mind to retain the logic pathways from which the selections are made, or the memory of the pathways chosen for individuals. Fortunately, because a machine can remember without fail and without distortion, accurate and complete records can be kept on individuals, and population studies can be done on their records.

From the purely scientific point of view, we are after statements that are precise and verifiable. As Karl Popper points out, the statement, "It will rain," is not very precise or testable as it does not deal with time, place, or circumstance; in contrast, the statement, "It will rain in London this afternoon," is verifiable, and for scientific purposes of feedback loop far more useful.[3] It is true that there is less probability of the latter statement being true than the broad statement, "It will rain"—the higher the information content, the lower the probability of occurrence. But to say less probability is another way of saying there are more ways the statement can be wrong. We are after statements, as Bryan Magee states in his book on Popper,[4] of high information content, therefore of low probability, which at the same time can come close to the truth. But we are safe, because the fact that such statements are highly falsifiable makes them maximally testable. To bring medicine's statements to as much precision as possible, and still not lose control of the extensive detail and branching logic, requires more than papers, pencils, and human minds. The computer becomes essential if intelligent application of expanding knowledge is ever to be a reality.

Our desire for maximum information has revealed increasing uniqueness among individuals, allowing us to meet their needs in more and more precise ways. But if we let the process of continuous elaboration occur, uncoupled to logical structures and separated from the largest possible universe of a given individual's concerns, we get lost in details, unable to return successfully to the larger purpose for which the pursuit was intended. That is precisely what has happened in medical education—details have been pursued out of all proportion to the pursuit of a structure in which to place them, give them meaning, and subject their application to control for the sake of the human individual in medical care.

The computer allows us to have the best of both context and content, if we use it as a tool and not place human minds in competition with its particular powers. It is no disgrace to our muscles to extend their function with automobiles, airplanes, spinning wheels, and surgeon's knives—we should therefore not shrink from extending our minds with computers, whose capabilities in areas of content retrieval in the proper context go beyond our own. This is not always easy to do in a society preoccupied with personal fulfillment and "independence" of all types. Interdependence, however, is a hallmark of highly developed civilizations—no one is complete unto himself, and personal fulfillment that requires this is an illusion that leads to frustration for individuals and trouble for those whom they purport to serve.

Our fulfillment must come from focusing on achieving the meaningful whole—like the performance of the system—and that in turn must come from using the tools around us instead of fearing them. Fear leads one to perceive structures on which one can build as merely constraints under which one must suffer. It is not surprising that many physicians have such fears, since their entire medical education was devoted to learning specialized aggregates of information and acting without rigorous feedback loops, as opposed to building structures, coordinating efforts, and analyzing results.

Medical schools, in particular, should stop trying to educate "the doctor," and instead educate a member of a team whose goal is clear. They should train him as a user of tools of communication adequate to the profession. Each medical provider should carve out that portion of the total job commensurate with his capabilities, prevent dependency states within it, be quick to recognize the limits of his capabilities, and then couple himself to the whole. Present memory-based medical education and examining procedures, and the mistaking of verbal and scribbled improvisations for a high form of medical art, preclude reliable feedback loops. They lead to a strange mixture of illusions of personal power and a crippling dependency on teachers and consultants, instead of to an understanding and utilization of good tools.

The function of medical education should be to help students define the borders of the areas in which they can perform reliably on their own. It should, furthermore, provide the tools and understanding whereby students couple their work to that of others at those borders. Faculties must recognize that for each student the area to be covered, and its boundaries, will be different—committees for providing for family practice and specialty programs, notwithstanding. No student or patient should ever function blindly under direction; he should function to fulfill a role and the responsibilities he clearly understands within the total.

The dependency states we want to avoid can be defined as those in which we function without knowing why, or do less than we reliably can in activities where we could solve problems on our own. This does not mean we should have total independence of tools or other human beings, for in a civilized society that is not achievable. We are in trouble in all areas of society because we create expectations and desires for independence, when interdependence and cooperation are both rewarding and necessary. And we unwittingly foster dependency states, whereas independence and responsibility are fulfilling as well as fundamental to preserving order. This happens in uncoupled systems. Medical education is no exception, and may even be an increasingly extreme example of uncoupling and waste.

There are those who fear that to tightly couple a human mind to computerized logic pathways, which that particular mind did not itself conceive, may destroy the spirit of inquiry and creativity. Such a fear suggests that because we acquire or use some knowledge by way of logical pathways described by others, we are not free to uncouple that knowledge from its pathway in our mind and apply it to create new pathways. Knowledge rarely comes to anyone completely disembodied from all problems and logic. In the computerized POMR the logic is always known at each step, and is designed to be related to the patient's needs, since it is his problems and all other recorded facts that selectively lead us through the pathways. No medical school ever passed out lists of facts independent of any logic in the mind of the lecturer or the textbook writer, and yet we do not fear destruction of inquiry by this stifling process of listening to lecturers. Our first responsibility is to couple knowledge to our patient's problems as tightly as possible. After that responsibility has been carried out, the student is free within his own personal "knowing structure," to use Piaget's term, to be as creative as he chooses with the information he has acquired as a by-product of useful work. At any rate, "type-ins" * are available at every step in the computer, and the user is always free to exercise his own logic in care, but never in ignorance of the foundation created by men of greater experience and expertise, and never free of accountability at precisely the point when the known logic was ignored and the improvisation of the user took over (Figure 5).

*   *   *   *

Having developed the role of the computer and the philosophical basis for proceeding with it, let us now review what that development requires as tasks are assigned to the computer that formally were assumed to be done by the human mind or were neglected altogether. Such a review can help crystallize new thoughts about teaching and the use and misuse of the human mind.

The basis of the system from the user's point of view is to make choices from a TV-like screen, and each choice either stores or merely brings forward another logically linked display from which storage, retrieval of information, or action may result. Since the words we read on a display are not written by human hands directed by some poorly understood human mechanism for memory, but rather are retrieved from a "disk" (computer memory-storage device) in which they are stored in electronic form, there must be some way of treating these displays as logical units and converting them to something that can be stored on a magnetic disk.

It is somewhat like interacting with a large library: you go there with a choice and must interact with its complicated mechanism and structures. The particular fact you want does not appear at the front door to greet you; there is a series of physical entities you or some-

---

* On all displays, where it is appropriate there is a choice "type-in." The user touches it and a blank screen appears on which he can type his own words.

THE OLD ROUTE:

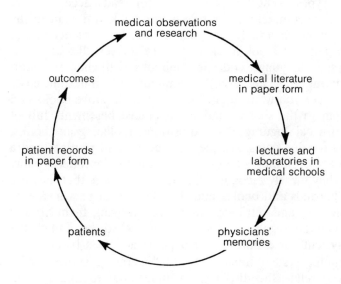

THE NEW ROUTE:

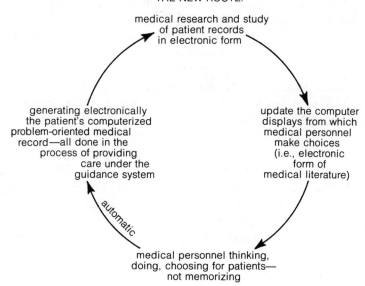

Figure 5. The Old Route and the New Route with the Computerized POMR.

one must understand in order to get to what you want. There are shelves of all types, some far away, some for ready access. There are card catalogues matching the title of the book you want to the language of numbers and letters that define the contents of the shelves; librarians who look in catalogues to correct titles and convert them to shelf language; codes in the books, with chapters, numbers, pages, paragraphs, and even line numbers, which in some cases lead you to where you want to go; loading carts to move books and to return them to the shelves and file cabinets; basements full of mechanisms for cataloguing new acquisitions, replacing lost books, and checking for due dates. All these structures and routines and a library language of numbers and letters are built independent of any given book; they merely recognize that there are facts, that they are kept within journals and books, and that there must be a means of acquiring, storing, and retrieving them, and moving them around efficiently. The aggregate of these means could be called the "operating system" of a library—or a pharmacy or a bank.

Our computer system must have an "operating system" with languages that relate the displays we understand to that system, languages that must represent a whole series of commands the "operating system" will execute, even if the user of the language is unaware of this. Furthermore, things must be so well-organized that responses will come within a quarter to a half a second, and they must be accurate—one false connection at any one of a thousand branch points among thousands of displays could lead to a senseless or even dangerous series of events.

Each touch of a display may not say directly where to go for a single retrieval. It may state in English, for example, that if a patient's blood pressure is above a certain level, proceed to such and such an order. The system must be able to search patient's records for specific facts, and then having done so and compared them proceed elsewhere to get the appropriate display in terms of what has "just been found" in the record. This means "searches" of "codes," which are in electronic form and part of the patient's electronic record. Multiple users of the terminals means sharing the system's resources and waiting in line, but never more than seconds, and never being forgotten and left hanging because the ideas somehow got lost in the system.

Before the computer, no one expected human beings at every single decision point to go to libraries, laboratories, pharmacies, and patients' records to retrieve relevant data according to logic pathways thought through by experts; most people could never understand each possible resource well enough to do that. And no one, of course, could ever do it with unfailing reliability in a quarter of a second. And so we chose to file as much information in the human mind as possible and use that operating system, which does work at remarkable speed. But, since the details of our human "computer" are unknown to us—and the relatively crude things that are known by psychologists are unknown to the average teacher of medicine— we treated the students' and doctors' minds as black boxes with some sort of shelves for storage, and hoped for the best. Occasionally we would give examinations to take inventory of what was on the shelves, and just assumed that if it were there it would be processed properly and in context. We focused on the content of the material on the shelves of the mind and did little to understand and to mold good "operating systems" independent of content.

Even assuming the human mind was as vast, reliable, and non-distorting as the computer, how often does it say, "I'll think about that and come back to it," and then let it be lost forever. How well does it handle interruptions, set priorities, and keep the proper items on the reserve shelf for immediate access? How carefully does it file all its experiences with consistent code numbers that allow immediate searches, and comparisons with searches of other human beings? What if we all have different operating systems, as we do different muscles and eyes and musical abilities? What are the implications of that for ways we handle information that medical faculties dispense? And if we handle things differently, as we treat disease, what are the implications for coordinating our thoughts with others and getting feedback loops on populations of people? And what are the implications for teaching? Should we be dealing more with the intellectual habits of people regardless of content—their capacity to be thorough and reliable, to think straight, and be efficient—in other words, working on the "operating systems" of human beings—how they handle tasks, deal with interruptions, file data in their minds, and deal with overloads? And should we be asking what sort of response times do people have, and what makes them "hang," and what makes them stop functioning altogether? Finally, the most disturbing thought of all concerns the development of human "operating systems." Are we born with a given one, or is it something that develops through usage, and, if so, how can that development be affected by educational practice, good and bad? The paper on medical education by George Nelson and his collaborators should be read or reread with these thoughts in mind.[5]

It doesn't help the patient to say we do not understand the mind that well, that all students will spend four years in medical school, and that at one point we shall merely see what is in their memory shelves and give them an *A, B,* or *C.* The patient, if he knew what was going on, would want to couple those student minds to operating systems we do understand and leave as little to educational roulette as possible. It is not surprising that our studies of errors in medicine reveal that only a rare error is based on the lack of availability of the right information—the bad mistakes are based on failure to review the information, or on hastily improvised and illogically arranged applications of facts randomly recalled by superficially informed generalists, or by specialists with great skill but a limited view of the patient's total needs. Furthermore, errors are based on poor systems and the lack of organization of tasks and responsibilities.

It is true that generalists and specialists may still ignore information, improvise, or continue to be provincial, even though we have computers. Two new factors are introduced, however, that our experiences suggests may and indeed have had a major effect. First, in the computer the facts are not only immediately available but tightly coupled to logic pathways for their application in the context of all pertinent information on the patient; many systems problems dealing with pharmacies, laboratories, etc. are thereby solved. Second, the removal of dependence on factual recall and the ready availability of information in logical form has enhanced the role of nurses and all other personnel to a significant degree. Their close relationship to and continuous presence among patients on a daily basis, doing the everyday work of medicine, allow them to put the newly available information to work in many and creative ways. The political implications of this for the role and rewards of physicians are enormous, and are just beginning to be felt. Medical educators must recognize these issues and act wisely on the patients' behalf. It is not their job to be loyal to any particular traditional role of the "doctor."

In discussing how the computer can assume such an important role, I should mention briefly how Jan Schultz, as a logical thinker trained in mathematics and logic and experienced with computers, began several years ago to develop a new language to deal with displays and the computerization of the POMR; thousands of those displays and structures were built by George Nelson, and his many collaborators. Ron Holland, Stu Graves, and Pete Walton further elaborated the structures as they, too, added content: a simple examination of a decision table for urinary tract infection will give some insight into the detail and structures that were required. Other individuals went through a whole set of processes in order to understand the operating system of a given computer, to modify it, and to develop languages so they could take the problem-oriented structure and the content developed by the medical group and create a functioning extension of the human mind. Steve Cantrill had to probe and unravel the details of how pharmacies, business offices, laboratories, and radiology departments operate in order to help incorporate their functions into a smoothly running coordinated medical care system.

From one point of view the system should be reviewed by others if for no other purpose than to show the massive complexity required to handle biological information with control and feedback, so that we might reflect on how badly we may have erred in "education" and in "using" the "human operating system." The Problem-Directed and Medical Information System (PROMIS), with its many complexities and moving parts, would be as mysterious to most people as the mind is to others from the outside. Study of the documentation is possible and rewarding, but, even more important, as it handles our information we get some idea of how faithful it is to good standards, whereas we still do not know how the human mind operates, or how similar each human bit of hardware is to another, and by not knowing we make serious assumptions in the practice of medicine.

As one reviews the hardware and software that the PROMIS group began with, that is, the control data equipment and its maintenance by Ernie Preiss, the ideas and languages of Robert Masters and Harlan Fretheim, and the creative efforts of Jim Wanner and others in developing new hardware and facilitating our conversion to Varian equipment from control data equipment, one realizes the crucial role of the materials with which one begins the task. All the dedication and genius in the world cannot overcome inadequate materials—even Beethoven could not perform his sonatas on a piano with twenty keys, a cracked sounding board, and strings that broke after the first fortissimo. We might barely sense that he was a potentially good composer and fine pianist, but that is all.

And, finally, over the years there have to be individuals with minds that understand what we are trying to do, and skills to see that displays are precisely written—logic pathways faithfully preserved with the tools at hand—and administrative relationships kept under control. Diane McGee has done that, and, although she has had help from many, her dedication from the beginning has made the difference. David Miller, an experienced health care administrator, has given essential administrative guidance in an almost unlimited number of ways.

Perhaps the most significant observation of all is that the computer, a powerful tool and an extension of the human mind, was absolutely essential to the integration of the efforts just described. Each group had to work through the computer or not at all: in this way it forced all activities to be coupled and cumulative or to come to a halt. The unregulated and uncoordinated proliferation of medical parts is not possible in such an environment. A computer system that works forces us to recognize interdependence among individuals' efforts, as well as the requirement that each individual be an independent thinker and reliable performer in the part of the whole in which he functions.

There might be some debate as to whether, for the everyday practice of medicine, medical faculties should fill students' minds with detailed descriptions of DNA or the Krebs cycle. There seems to be less and less doubt, however, that we must reassess what we have expected of the human mind, and what tools are available to support it, when the specifications of human capabilities are not up to the functions we need to carry out. We quickly give mechanical support to muscles when functions require it.

We have used technology to extend the senses to a far greater degree than most physicians articulate or even realize. Techniques with sound waves applied over many parts of the body, catheters, X-rays, amplification, and analysis of all sorts of electrical phenomena from the body—all go well beyond the unaided hand, eye, and ear. And now these techniques are being coupled to the computer, thereby increasing their power of resolution many-fold. Although the original X-ray was far better than human vision for many lesions in the body, for example, it was limited by current photographic techniques and subtle changes in density were lost. This has now been altered by the use of new techniques to determine directly thousands of gradations in the transmission of X-rays, and the ability to deal with the large amount of data generated by coupling to the computer. The same coupling can and has been done with sound waves. Having "digitized" the data for computer analysis and subsequent presentation of "patterns" for us to view, not only can the surgical operation or autopsy "teach" us what the patterns mean, it can give direct and specific diagnostic meaning to the data residing in the computer, independent of conversion to the typical "photographic-like" pattern familiar to us.

As far greater quantities of data from each part of the human system are more and more precisely defined and computerized, it becomes ever more urgent to coordinate the use of that data for the benefit of the whole individual and of society. As pointed out earlier, such coordination and rigorous feedback loops require the computer. We must overcome our tendency to recapitulate old methods and old notions, instead of leapfrogging over them, particularly the notion that the unaided human mind and senses are the best instruments for deciding which data to acquire, for routinely acquiring data, and for processing data once they are obtained. To the extent that our instruments and computers are limited in these processes, the human mind is often even more limited.

It is true that the computer needs to be programmed on the basis of reliable data in the right context, but so does the mind. In this regard the mind frequently and recklessly embarks on the impossible task of trying to recall and assemble the proper data from fallible human memories, and then proceeds from one step to the next by processes unknown to others and even to the individual thinker himself. Certainly no one believes that the mind is systematically introducing one variable at a time, doing calculations at lightening speed using Bayes theorem or other techniques. In contrast, when using the computer guidance system described earlier, data are requested according to previously developed logic, and the computer can reliably search among already computerized data on an individual as computerized decision tables require it. The relatively incomplete decision tables we now have, because of poor medical records, can be updated and improved in the future from accumulated computer data, using the appropriate mathematical techniques to allow the maximal yield from a minimal amount of data economically acquired. It is pointless to bemoan our ignorance and say we do not yet know enough to program the computer. We never will know enough if we do not start, make first approximations using present knowledge and structured input, analyze our results, update our pathways, and bootstrap our way up. We should have started long ago—but never mind, let us get on with it. The studies that have been made simply do not bear out the notion that the human mind when unaided is up to the task.[6] The mind is willing to proceed without adequate data and feedback loops, and, having done so, is much more apt to conclude it was correct without the evidence, that is, clinical judgment is the willingness to make decisions on inadequate data.

If it is a myth that the mind uses properly all the data available to it and rigorously applies that portion of the data it does use, then what is the role of the human mind? It is to build the structures and the appropriate hardware and software that can supersede the mind's own unaided performance in the routine use of large amounts of data. This is not a trivial task, but it does alter dramatically, and in many cases simply supplants, the traditional role of physicians in the routine practice of medicine when it involves the rigorous analysis of large amounts of data—that is, the daily application of medical science to human needs. As A. N. Whitehead has stated:

> It is a profoundly erroneous truism, repeated by all copy-books and by eminent people when they are making speeches, that we should cultivate the habit of thinking about what we are doing. The precise opposite is the case. Civilization advances by extending the number of important operations which we can perform without thinking about them. Operations of thought are like cavalry charges in a battle—they are strictly limited in number, they require fresh horses, and must only be made at decisive moments.[7]

We have only barely begun to exploit the enormous capabilities for manipulating complex data structures in a highly interactive computer terminal environment. It is to this area that the efforts of the PROMIS laboratory are being directed within the framework of the problem-oriented philosophy for comprehensive care. The question should never be minds or computers, but rather what is the most effective combination for getting the job done. As we stated in 1969:

> All of us would like to correct this imbalance, to see the organization of medicine well studied and well ordered, without, at the same time, shifting the weight of research and planning so far that the undeniable benefits of a concentration on specialized subject areas are lost. Indeed, not only would the standard of medical care aspired to in this volume be impossible without medicine's long history of the closely focused and theoretical study of the science of health and disease, but it is precisely in the effort to apply the fruits of that research effectively and

broadly and to order and integrate the elements of it that this volume has been prepared.[8]

It is true that there is such a thing as the "placebo effect," that is, unknown forces are released in a patient to help him do better if he thinks he is being helped, even if there is no rigorous evidence that the therapy applied is sound. In this sense physicians could outdo computers in environments where computers are downgraded and physicians deified. But the reverse would be true in situations where a computer is more trusted to deal with a complex situation than an unaided mind. The public will want the best possible combination of the two once they begin to understand the present problems of coordination and broken feedback loops in the everyday practice of medicine. Magnificent isolated achievements in medical specialties do not relieve us of the social responsibility for meaningful comprehensive care or the scientific responsibility for understanding the relationships among the parts as well as the specialized parts themselves.

Whether the positions stated here can be supported by medical faculties and whether they in time will be implemented in medical schools are questions that many medical students of today have to struggle with.

NEW AND OLD PREMISES FOR MEDICAL EDUCATION

In the first section we discussed the structure of the present medical care and education system. Certain flaws in this structure were analyzed on the basis of what we know about capabilities of the human mind and limitations of the communications systems now in use. The second section described two tools to deal with these problems—the manual POMR and computerized POMR. The philosophical basis for shifting to such tools was also presented.

These new tools extend, amplify, and alter the role of the human mind in medical care activities. They thereby lead to reassessment of the very premises on which medical education is based. I shall first review the old premise, then present the new, and, finally, state specifically how the new tools and the new premises combine to allow practical implementation of a medical curriculum.

Memory

> Old Premise: A core of knowledge should be taught.
> New Premise: A core of behavior should be elicited.

Regardless of what we might say about our philosophy of education, our examination structure gives us away. We examine students and practicing physicians for what they know in terms of medical facts. Sometimes in these examinations we ask them to reason logically with what they know, but nevertheless they are expected to carry a core of knowledge with them.

What has this led to? First, it has probably catalyzed specialization, since if one is going to be examined on what one knows one must narrow the field down in order to pass examinations in a world of such rapidly expanding knowledge. At the time this process is going on, the patient as an organism cannot of course specialize, and the problem of coordinated care is exacerbated. The mere institution of family practice programs may not help the situation if the basic premise is unchanged, since it does not recognize the forces that led to the loss of family practitioners in the first place.

Second, the "memory," "core-of-knowledge" approach led to a mentality in medicine that not only thought it could memorize information it would need for practice, but that it could carry in the mind much information about the patients themselves. It allowed physicians to keep records in which they did not feel it necessary in their plans and progress notes to preserve their logic on a day-to-day basis, since they believed they could remember it. They presumably could always remember "why," if evidence of the order or act were preserved. It led physicians to think of themselves as "the physician" instead of as members of a medical team, using a well-thought-out communications system to protect patients when medical personnel went on vacation, took evenings off, or went into a speciality.

A core-of-knowledge approach allowed us to think that the student's mind was so good that we could give him two years of answers in the so-called basic science years before we told him the questions. Implicit in all this was the assumption that he would slowly see the whole of medical care on his own, and would remember enough facts about enough people to provide a statistically significant feedback loop for correction of medical action. Many of our difficulties have their roots in our premises about the role of the human memory and the teaching of the core of knowledge.

Our new premise should be to elicit a core of behavior rather than a core of knowledge, and never examine for or actively memorize knowledge. We should recognize the fact that memory is usage— not IQ, not interest, but usage. Use a thing or do an act over and over and one automatically comes to know it. Memorize something and then fail to use it and it will escape the memory when you need it. There are those who say, "But there are certain basic things one needs to know by heart before one can practice." It is a myth that we ever allowed any student on the basis of his memorized knowledge to treat, for the first time, a ventricular tachycardia or any other medical problem in an emergency from that memorized base alone. He has always been asked to work with others and watch a few treatments before he does it alone. In those nonemergency situations the student always has time to look things up, and it is amazing how effective he can become at this, given a little practice. The emphasis should be on eliciting a core of behavior, that is, thoroughness, reliability, a sound analytic sense, and efficiency.[9]

Acceptance of this new premise means we must abolish the national board examinations as we now know them, and look in an unannounced random manner at how people perform in the real world according to a core of behavior. This can and has been done, and could be developed on a nation-wide basis if it were our will to do so.

The Resources and Capital Investment of a Medical School

Old Premise: *Faculty, research facilities, specialized extensive clinical facilities, and teaching facilities are the principal resources of a medical school.*

New Premise: *The principal resource of a medical school is the student's natural capacity to learn on his own and solve problems on his own in an environment that allows and encourages him to do so, and provides essential feedback.*

Although not always stated explicitly, it is an underlying premise of modern medical schools that they require a huge capital investment, with extensive research laboratories, large numbers of specialized faculty, and multimillion dollar budgets. This, for the most part, grows out of the old premise. When one focuses on knowledge to the exclusion of other things, one is forced to overemphasize educational facilities that produce new knowledge and encourage attempts to transmit memorized knowledge. It is of course appropriate that we have research institutes for the accumulation of new medical information, but if they are properly organized, and if students learn a significant core of behavior, the cost of medical research need not be charged to medical education. Because we have considered these large investments as a fundamental resource, we are pricing medical education out of the reach of a great many citizens we would most like to have it, and who are best equipped to provide care to large segments of the population.

The new premise should be that the greatest resource of the medical school is the student's capacity to solve problems on his own, using every tool, new and old, available to him. The function of the school should be to emphasize and develop that capacity, so that instead of breeding people who need more and more intellectual diaper-changing and postgraduate education, we have individuals with resourceful, independent minds who will naturally turn to books and modern computer techniques and all the other sources of information and skills that abound in our society, independent of the formal development and expenses of a medical school and its faculty.

The consequences of a new premise in this area may be far-reaching indeed. The medical schools create intellectual dependency states in their students, who, when they become doctors, in turn create dependency states in their patients. Furthermore, medical students develop a complete misconception of the doctor-patient relationship and of their role as a member of a medical team.

The whole matter of dependency states should perhaps be elaborated here, since not only is the student's capacity to solve problems on his own a great untapped resource of the medical schools, but a patient's capacity to do things for himself is the biggest untapped resource in the medical care system. The development of these resources is closely related. The doctor-patient and teacher-student relationships should be thought of as guide and auditor-performer relationships; the present unacceptable reality is performer-object relationship. Both patient and students must become active instead of passive, and these new premises, new curriculum, and the new book for patients, *Your Health Care and How to Manage It,*[10] are directed toward this goal. Medical students should not be educated to believe that their emotional involvement with patients differs from that of any other practitioner of the medical arts.*

---

* It is unfortunate that the word "patient" is so deeply embedded in our culture. Historically and at present it reflects the exploitation and paternalism one sees in the medical care system. Ivan Illich is not wholly unjustified in the devastating use of the phrase "expropriation of health."[11] In the dictionary, the word "patient" as a noun is defined as one "receiving care or treatment . . .

It should be a conscious goal of an organization for medical care to avoid the principal pitfall of the old doctor-patient relationship—the dependency states of patients on any single individual provider. Patients should be taught about the whole system and encouraged to exercise maximum independence, so they do not become victims of the unrealistic demands for availability of personnel and resources that their dependency state implies.

Far more medical actions now considered to require a trained physician can actually be performed well by people who have not had extensive physician training—if the right tools are provided and if the points made here are understood and accepted.

When physicians' economic rewards greatly exceed those of others in the system, they should receive these rewards only for tasks that are unique to them through training that was unique, necessary, and expensive—not through some rites of passage that are either out of date or ill-conceived in the first place. No system should start out with the serious financial constraint of large salaries for the M.D. unless a careful analysis of his work can justify them.

A main goal of university medicine should be, wherever possible, to transfer tasks to less expensive personnel, to encourage independence and responsibility in patients, and to develop and foster the use of new tools that will promote efficiency. We certainly should not reward those whose methods prevent the extension of medicine to large numbers of people at low cost, and who, by their concept of the doctor-patient relationship, create dependency states in patients, which in the long-run are not only bad for doctors and patients alike, but economically disastrous for society as a whole.

Our present medical structure cannot be extended to all the people, given our current financial resources and tools. Acceptance of the foregoing points and the rapid development of new tools, including the computer, are therefore necessary.

The points just stated apply directly to the relationship between teacher and students. The focus should not be on taking something away from physicians or teachers and their particular happy group of patients or students. Indeed one can feel nothing but sympathy for a physician or a teacher who is trapped with beliefs about

---

capable of bearing (fatigue, thirst, etc.)." Directly above is the definition of the adjective: "bearing or enduring pain, trouble, etc. without complaining, losing self-control . . . refusing to be provoked or angered, as by an insult; forbearing, tolerant . . . calmly tolerating delay, confusion, inefficiency, etc." These very definitions provide the wrong context for the constructive changes now needed in medical practice.

methodology that make his efforts far less meaningful than they could be to large numbers of patients or students.

Robert H. Moser states that, "I cherish the opportunity to speak to *my* patients." [12] The assertions in the foregoing pages deal with the majority of patients, even Moser's patients, who are not "cherished" by anyone when the physician is on vacation, or dies, or decides he no longer wants to treat a patient who has a problem outside of his specialty or area of interest, or on his night off, or in his month "off-service" in an academic setting.

At a time when the medical profession has demonstrated incontrovertibly that it cannot do everything with its present methodologies and training programs, it should not with selfish nostalgia prevent the progress of those who could and want to help with new tools and far less expensive training. Not only is it unfair to the patients no one sees, it is tragic for those in whom doctors create a dependency state and then, without warning or preparation, suddenly retire or take a hospital job, administrative position, or academic role with few direct patient care responsibilities. This could all be avoided if we admitted in the first place that we must rethink the phrase "doctor-patient relationship," as well as medical education itself.

A typical example of fostering an unnecessary dependency state between student and teacher is when the latter reviews a case with a new clinical clerk and discovers the student has performed poorly in 80 percent of his efforts, but quite adequately in the other 20 percent. He usually proceeds to teach and give information in the area of deficiency. Frequently, however, if he investigates the matter, he may find the 20 percent done correctly was the result of the student's initiative and pursuit of the correct information. He should recognize this, encourage the student to pursue the other 80 percent in a similar fashion, and thereby cultivate intellectual independence. Our present approaches keep inculcating the notion that in order to learn something you have to be taught.

Because we have failed to identify the true fundamental resources of the medical school, we have prevented the development of less expensive medical schools, as well as regional schools that would support candidates indigenous to those areas. We have also by the same mechanism fostered the specialization and growth of numbers of faculty members within medical school departments well beyond the stage where this is productive for individual students. As a matter of fact it has probably interfered with the proper development of the students' basic habits and conceptual development concerning all of medicine. The whole system whereby medical schools are approved and accredited needs to be reconsidered and set on a different course.

Real Work and Responsibility

> *Old Premise: Students should learn given facts and understanding in the absence of real work and real responsibility.*
> *New Premise: Real work with real responsibilities should should form the basis of all educational activity right from the beginning.*

For many years medical students, at least in their first two years of medical school, have been engaged in learning programs that do not involve real work. Frequently they are not even engaged in problem solving, and on those occasions when they are, they deal with problems to which the solutions are already known. In such a situation it is difficult to teach responsibility. A student may not feel irresponsible if he fails to do what he considers a teacher's busy work. But it is a rare student who, having agreed to do real work for patients in his chosen profession, would deny he is being irresponsible when he does not make a sincere attempt to get the work done.

It is a misconception to think that real work or so-called applied science cuts the student off from theoretical development. Tolstoy warned us against the snare of preparation that members of various disciplines insist on imposing upon students before they let them do real work. We should be reminded, as Popper said, that:

> Disciplines are distinguished partly for historical reasons and reasons of administrative convenience (such as the organization of teaching and of appointments), and partly because the theories which we construct to solve our problems have a tendency to grow into unified systems. But all this classification and distinction is a comparatively unimportant and superficial affair. We are not students of some subject matter but students of problems. And problems may cut right across the borders of any subject matter or discipline.[13]

The teacher's job is to pick problems appropriate to a student's level; there are many in medicine that they can start with at the very beginning.

When a student fails to deal with real problems effectively, it is the faculty's job to find out why. Are his cognitive skills poorly developed? Can't he read or find facts? Can't he synthesize them after comprehending them? Can't he apply them or evaluate the results of his application? Or is his problem one of attitude and affect? Is he not interested in the work? Or can't he deal effectively with other people in getting the job done? Or perhaps he has trouble with manipulative skills, on which he is dependent at some stage of solving a problem. Real problems, properly pursued as we elicit a core of behavior, automatically lead us to the so-called noncognitive areas in education and evaluation.

How sad it is when we cannot be creative and imaginative enough to find real problems appropriate to the student's stage of development, and impose on him instead, in Popper's words:

> . . . a world of astonishingly subtle and vast abstractions. Thoughts and arguments are put before the student's mind which sometimes are not only hard to understand but which seem to him irrelevant because he cannot find out what they may be relevant to. But some students will say to themselves that this must be the way of medicine and will make an effort to adjust the mind to what he believes (mistakingly as we shall see) to be another's way of thinking. He will attempt to speak their language, to match the tortuous spirals of his teacher's argumentation and perhaps even tie himself up in the teacher's curious knots. Some may learn tricks in a superficial way and others may begin to become genuinely fascinated addicts.[14]

But there are other students who will not make such an effort and who will leave medicine. With our present premises we may have unwittingly found a way to select against the problem solvers, who will accept the challenges of any environment they find themselves in and rejoice in the opportunity to confront real problems, happy to get the world's work done, and confident that, in such efforts, their imaginations will be challenged and theoretical implications will flow in their minds from what outwardly appear to be trivial indeed. Creative people turn to nature and real things, not to schoolrooms.

Time and Number of Tasks

Old Premise: Time and number of courses covered should be the constant, and achievement the variable in medical education.

*New Premise: Achievement should be the constant, and
time and number of tasks the variable in
medical education and medical practice.*

At the present time in medical education we make time and the
number of tasks the constant, and the level of achievement the
variable. Every student takes biochemistry or cardiology in the same
amount of time, and at the end we give some an *A*, some a *B*, some
a *C*, and flunk others. We have almost developed a way to institu-
tionalize the teaching of mediocrity and sloppiness. If our goal had
been to elicit a core of behavior—thoroughness, reliability, sound
analytical sense, and efficiency—instead of a core of knowledge,
and if we had been dealing with real work, it would not have been
so easy to fall into this trap. In athletics it is not so simple, because
on a ski slope equal training time regardless of the natural talent of
individuals, results in more than *As* and *Bs* and *Cs*—it results in
broken legs and the abandonment of skiing as a pleasurable sport
by many people who under different circumstances could have done
well and enjoyed it immensely.

There are many ways to make achievement the constant, and time
and number of tasks the variable for the benefit of society, but it is
doubtful that this will be done by medical school administrators who
are prisoners of the old premises. Many present leaders are hard-
working, honest people with great management talents who do a
magnificent job within the premises they have accepted. But the
question is, are we dealing with successful navigation to the wrong
port—pride in setting and achieving one set of educational objectives, but totally unconscious of another whole world of objectives
that might be far more meaningful to students and patients alike in
the long run.

Credentials

*Old Premise: A person should take examinations such
as national boards and specialty boards at
one point in his education in order to
qualify for practice.*

*New Premise: A person's performance should be audited
at random throughout his career, and, according to rules for medical practice,
clearly defined and used from the very
beginning of medical education.*

At the present time an M.D. degree and a license to practice are awarded after a fixed time of formal education based on examinations given at a certain point on a core of knowledge and some analytical techniques. Medical students assume that this degree carries with it, in addition to the opportunity to practice, a certain place on the medical team, future financial rewards, and a level of prestige second to none in the medical hierarchy. Most students are not aware historically of how the present situation of physicians developed. They are apt to assume a security in the doctor's position that may not in fact be justified. Certainly most medical students do not feel any obligation to reassess the position of doctors in society with a view to making readjustments in the light of new tools and new approaches to patient care.

In the new situation, credentials should be based on performance, randomly audited over a lifetime. This is precisely what is done with investigators in all areas, as they submit each new piece of work for review, regardless of who they are, where they trained, or how many papers they have published. Nothing short of observing work being done in the actual environment in which a person is expected to function can predict future performance. It follows naturally from this premise that, with performance as the standard, many people with natural talents and new tools may reach high levels of performance without some of the so-called "preparation" that a credential-oriented society tends to foster.

Perhaps the most useful thing medical educators can do for medical and premedical students is to proclaim that the definitions, the role, and the rewards of a physician are changing so fast that he should not be surprised at any turn of events. Nothing can be guaranteed except the chance to explore, to question, and to contribute to the changing field of medicine. And, finally, educators should provide an environment in which everyone welcomes the skills and insights of individuals of diverse and nontraditional backgrounds.

THE POMR IN RELATIONSHIP TO THE NEW PREMISES

Eliciting a Core of Behavior

The rules of the POMR allow us to focus completely on whether the student is thorough, reliable, analytically sound, and efficient—that is, on his core of behavior. He is never ashamed to use the record as an extension of his mind. The focus shifts from his capacity to dazzle people with isolated bits of recalled knowledge of both the literature and his patients to his capacity to always be thorough and logical in an open manner that can be easily understood and checked by the patients. The POMR facilitates the development of teachers who are auditors rather than transmitters of information. Normally the traits of thoroughness, reliability, analytical sense, and efficiency sound like vague platitudes, but with the problem-oriented record they suddenly achieve very specific meaning. These traits can be assessed, elicited, and developed.[15]

The Principal Resource of a Medical School Is the Capacity of Students and Patients to Solve Problems on Their Own

The problem-oriented record provides a structure for any student to see immediately what it is we are trying to do in medical practice. Frequently students start off learning bits and pieces, accepting on faith that those pieces fit into the practice of medicine, the details of which they perceive only dimly. It is absolutely crucial that students first see the structure of what we are trying to do, so their own powers can be mobilized. Otherwise all they can develop is their memories, and memory hypertrophies out of all proportion to the development of other logical faculties. The record provides the only immunization the student has against the generalizations and misconceptions of those who would teach him. His ultimate teacher should be reality; the teacher should be an auditor who makes sure that there is absolute honesty, reliability, and sound thought as these realities in biology are faced. The teacher is not there to solve problems, but to see that the student does. The POMR is the means by which they communicate, and by which the students' ability to solve problems on his own is discerned and developed.

Real Work and Responsibility

The POMR is the tool whereby the large number of acts that make up total care can be divided into manageable and reasonable groups and still not lose their meaningful relationships to one another. The POMR allows each medical provider to be a member of a team that works logically and efficiently to solve problems. It allows for synthesis and the perception of new relationships among the elegant pieces of each specialist.

Since the POMR allows us to break up total care into parts without losing the sense of wholeness, we can make those parts as small as necessary for the beginning student and thereby start him with real work, whereby we can judge and teach responsibility, as well as purely technical and intellectual skills.

Credentials

With records that preserve logic immediately available, we can retrieve at any time the efforts of any provider in the system as we audit for quality. The person should be known by his performance; he should be in a position to be evaluated at any point in his career. This can be done if the results of his efforts are in electronic form and immediately available at any site. Many ways can be developed to look at his behavior at any given moment in terms of goals for patients, as opposed to outdated goals for disciplines independent of patients. A diploma of the bricks as opposed to the diploma of the books can truly become a reality.[16]

Structure

Is the medical system as we know it a true structure, or is it just an aggregate of conflicting interests presided over by leaders who articulate "caution" and the wisdom of living in the "real world" they inherited? Our recollection of the tenure of such leaders is often one of management of budgets and events that surround them, or of the fates of people they "hammer" into or out of place —forever seeking strength by political carpentry. Rarely do we see a leader seeking strength through the loud and clear articulation of an overall design for coordinating a system of health care, medical research, and medical education—a design which, if relentlessly pursued, would call into play the right pieces, regardless of past traditions, and reject those that would corrupt the overall goals for patients and society.

It is not enough for a leader to answer that he has a private vision: he must articulate it for two reasons. First, each of us can play his part well and with a sense of fulfillment only if he sees the whole slowly emerging before him; second, if there are flaws in the structure, others can see them and help correct them, otherwise we shall not have a true structure that, in Piaget's terms, contains within it the ideas of wholeness, of transformation, and of self-regulation. Rather, we shall merely revert to our present uncoupled medical care system and get lost among the disconnected pieces, rationalizing appeasement of autonomous groups as providing "incentives" based on political realities.

Our present data indicate that the distribution of surgery follows the distribution of surgeons more than need; the distribution of physicians in general follows the distribution of dollars more than need. Audit demonstrates that the best basic science teacher in the old paradigm may have transiently transmitted the facts of basic science, but the behavior of the scientist escaped many of his graduates. No overall architectural plan has been developed to control the random infiltration of the medical care system with all types of expensive and powerful technologies. It is unlikely that the present leaders of medicine and medical education, who have been brought up in the old paradigm and who have led us to where we are now, will come forth with new designs, accept new designs of others, or even admit that they are needed.

It is time now for each of us to think about the whole. If the design presented in the foregoing pages is sound, then to build up one part is to automatically tighten the whole structure and strengthen the others. The more we solve the coordination problem, the more complete the feedback; the more complete the feedback, the sounder the logic of future acts; the more demanding we are of the precise execution of logic pathways, the less memory-dependent the system must become. Or we can proceed in the reverse direction, tightening the structure each step of the way. The concepts described are given expression with the tools of the manual POMR and the computerized POMR. If we would have confidence in the strength of our design and articulate it to all, not just to the leaders of the old paradigm, then the design itself would lead us securely to rearrange resources, personnel, and rewards in a way that present leaders may never do.

The following words of Piaget take on more and more meaning for us now:

> . . . the pyramid of knowledge no longer rests on foundations, but hangs by its vertex, an ideal point never reached and more curious constantly rising! In short, rather than envisage human knowledge as a pyramid or building of some sort, we should think of it as a spiral, the radius of whose turns increases as the spiral rises.[17]

CONCLUSION

Many of the inadequacies of medical care have resulted from false premises in medical education and poor tools. Misconceptions about the capabilities of the human memory and failure to use modern communications tools in a meaningful way have allowed medical care, medical records, and medical education to become dangerously uncoupled. With almost infinite biological and social complexity to feed on, each has taken on a life of its own because they were not placed in structures that forced meaningful relationships and regulation among them. We never built the tool to unambiguously sort good medical actions from bad over a long period of time in the lives of individuals, and so medical education has been blind, unrealistic commitments have been made, and unrealizable expectations fostered; and medical research, which has been uncoupled in the larger context, has been more than willing to busy itself with the infinite elaboration of details.

New premises and new tools are available whereby we can discover where we are and where we are going, but they offer no assurance that we shall change our course. Medical education above all else should now teach students that as we begin the process of applying new methods, roles formerly limited to a few will open to many. Long years of expensive and formal education are no justification of anything, especially if they do not serve the purposes intended. To the extent that students will be stimulated by the prospect of more care to more people with less elitism and paternalism among providers, they can improve the new tools and forge ahead, enjoying the future. To the extent that their future happiness is predicated on present hierarchies among providers, and high financial rewards for physicians relative to all others in the scheme, each should be prepared for frustrating struggles and disappointing defeats as they are overtaken by many others in society, including patients. The patients will gain understanding and authority from the applications of the new premises and new tools of communication.

The issues are clear and the new tools can become a reality for everyone. The decisions are now political, and the responsibility lies with the leaders in medicine and society in general.

Notes

1. Lawrence L. Weed, *Your Health Care and How to Manage It* (Essex Junction, Vermont: Essex Publishing Co., 1975).
2. For a more detailed description of the system see: J. E. Schultz, Stephen V. Cantrill, and Keith G. Morgan, "An Initial Operational Problem-Oriented Medical Record System—For Storage, Manipulation and Retrieval of Medi-

cal Data," *AFIPS-Conference Proceedings* 38 (1971): 239–64; see also: Weed, *Your Health Care,* chaps. 19 and 21 (see note 1).

3. Bryan Magee, *Karl Popper* (New York: Viking Press, 1973).

4. Ibid.

5. George Nelson et al., "A Performance-Based Method of Student Evaluation," *British Journal of Medical Education* 10 (1976): 33–42.

6. For example see: *Journal of the Royal College of Physicians of London* 9, no. 3 (April 1975): 191–278.

7. Alfred N. Whitehead, quoted by Christopher Strachey, "System Analysis in Programming," in *Computers and Computation Readings from Scientific American* (San Francisco: W. H. Freeman & Co., 1971).

8. Lawrence L. Weed, *Medical Records, Medical Education and Patient Care* (Cleveland, Ohio: Case Western Reserve University Press, 1969).

9. The details of eliciting these traits are discussed in: Nelson et al., "Method of Student Evaluation" (see note 5); see also: J. Willis Hurst and H. Kenneth Walker, *The Problem-Oriented System* (New York: Medcom, Inc., 1972): chaps. 11 and 14; and Weed, *Your Health Care* (see note 1).

10. Weed, *Your Health Care* (see note 1).

11. Ivan Illich, *Medical Nemesis* (London: Calder & Boyars, 1975).

12. Robert H. Moser, "The First Five Minutes," *Journal of the American Medical Association* 231, no. 1 (1975): 1169.

13. Magee, *Karl Popper* (see note 3).

14. Ibid.

15. Hurst and Walker, *Problem-Oriented System,* chap. 14 (see note 9); and Nelson et al., "Method of Student Evaluation" (see note 5).

16. Lawrence L. Weed, "A Touchstone for Medical Education," *Harvard Alumni Bulletin* (November/December 1974): 13–18.

17. Jean Piaget, *Structuralism* (New York: Basic Books, Inc., 1970).

DISCUSSION

In reply to a question about undue dependence on the computer, Weed replied that other tools—a stethoscope, electrocardiagraph, etc.—on which the physician relies do not constitute a form of dependence. If appropriate support is forthcoming, the computer too can be made readily available in all clinical situations. In the meantime, where it is not now available, the student can still transfer to the ward the mode of thought he was taught in the PROMIS program.

The Three-Year Curriculum: Advantages and Disadvantages

✿

ROBERT D. SPARKS, GUY T. HAVEN,
IRENE KLINTBERG, and PERRY G. RIGBY *

It is often helpful to contrast principles of education for health professionals with principles of education in other fields. Such a contrast offered itself during a recent flight through some mountainous terrain well known to some medical educators. A card in the seat-pocket of the aircraft flying into a resort area and conference center in the Rocky Mountains offered words intended to be reassuring to passengers on the flight. The need for such reassurance could, and does, cause some consternation among the passengers, in spite of the airline's best intentions. A reading of the message with slight paraphrasing could be applicable to the circumstances facing a new dean of a medical school. Imagine that the following edited message was prepared by the faculty of a medical school, rather than the management of an airline, as a greeting to the new dean, a special passenger, on his new flying venture as administrator. Finally, imagine the mountains to be the educational plan for the curriculum of the medical school. This rephrasing of the airline's message constitutes an appropriate setting for the report on the three-year curriculum that follows. The modified message reads:

Dear Mr. Dean:

You are about to have a unique sightseeing adventure. Your flight covers some of the most dramatic mountains [of medical education]

* Only Dr. Sparks attended the conference. His coauthors at the University of Nebraska Medical Center are: Dr. Haven, associate professor, Department of Pathology, research associate professor of biochemistry, and assistant dean for curriculum; Dr. Klintberg, assistant professor of medical and educational administration; and Dr. Rigby, professor, Department of Internal Medicine, and dean, College of Medicine.

in the country, and we will be flying at altitudes that enable you the best possible view. If you are not accustomed to flying the mountains [of medical education] you may be initially somewhat uneasy as the clear mountain air causes the scenery [of medical education] to appear much closer than it is.

The weather in the mountains [of medical education] moves very rapidly and is, at times, as dramatic as the scenery; consequently some of our flights are bumpy and a few are downright rough. This is no cause for alarm, but merely a typical condition when flying over the Rocky Mountains [of medical education].

In short, relax and enjoy your trip. We think it is the most spectacular flight in the country, and we, as the only scheduled [medical school] serving the mountains [of medical education] in these parts, know what we are doing.

Sincerely,
Your Faculty

*   *   *   *

The advantages and disadvantages of a three-year medical curriculum must be considered from the viewpoint of several categories of individuals or groups. These include the students enrolled in the educational program; the faculty who teach in it; the administration and board of the institution presenting the program; the public; and the peer group, in this instance the profession of medicine. Unfortunately statements of advantages and disadvantages too often must be subjective observations rather than objective conclusions.

A particular problem in addressing these advantages and disadvantages is the difficulty in defining precisely what is meant by a three-year curriculum. A comparison of such a curriculum in one medical school with another indicates that the educational program may follow traditional departmental lines or it may be dominated by interdepartmental and organ system presentations. The amount of emphasis placed on separate basic science courses, apart from clinical science education, varies considerably. Without careful examination it is often hard to define how a three-year curriculum differs from a former four-year program in the same school. Following such scrutiny it may be apparent that the only real distinction between the two is, in fact, the span of time alloted for completion of the same curriculum. Within a given institution a three-year curriculum for two succeeding classes may differ significantly. The changes result from decisions to alter it as a consequence of experiences in the previous year.

A major challenge is to define the intent of the "three-year" curriculum. In the case of medicine, clearly the purpose is to establish that the product, the physician, is a qualified professional who may or may not seek further education, but in either event will be prepared to give appropriate medical care in the role of an independent practitioner. (In some states, laws governing medical practice permit practice immediately after graduation from medical school without requiring further graduate education in an internship or residency.) The individual curriculum must be judged for quality, and, ideally, the quality desired should be defined in advance. Ultimately, the quality of the *product,* the medical graduate, becomes the challenge for judging the curriculum, although other subsidiary questions and goals do influence the categorization of observations. Certainly each institution has its own reasons for introducing a three-year course, and those reasons also help determine advantages and disadvantages. If one were to poll the several medical schools that have introduced three-year curricula, I am certain the subsidiary motiviations would vary considerably.

As of October 1975, nineteen medical schools in the United States offered a three-year curriculum as their *basic* educational program; * in 1973–74 only eleven schools required a three-year course of all students.[1] Many schools offering a four-year curriculum as a basic requirement do permit an optional accelerated program. In 1971–72, forty schools had an option to complete the curriculum in less than four years, whereas in 1973–74 the option was available in fifty-nine schools.[2]

As everyone in medical education is aware, in recent years there has been a phenomenal growth in the number of entering places in our medical schools—from approximately nine thousand matriculants in the mid-1960s to almost fifteen thousand in 1975.[3] According to data from the Association of American Medical Colleges (AAMC) there may be as many as eighteen or nineteen thousand new places by 1985, if current commitments for expansion are fulfilled.

The second major change since the early 1960s has been reexploration of the shortened period of time required for medical education. Those who wish to reflect on the elements that encouraged the expansion of enrollments and the shortened curriculum should

---

* Robert L. Beran, Ph.D., project coordinator for the three-year curriculum study of the Association of American Medical Colleges (National Institutes of Health contract): personal communication.

read John A.D. Cooper's 1971 paper, "External Forces Influencing Medical Education." [4] Of the several factors he mentions, it is noteworthy that in the early 1960s a major change in public pressure influenced medical education. The Congress of the United States enacted legislation that forced a significant shift in national purpose from support of biomedical research to assistance for medical education and an expansion of medical services to the elderly, to those with a few major categorical illnesses, and to the economically disadvantaged. In 1963 it passed the Health Professions Education Assistance Act, which initiated the current programs that provide major financial assistance to American medical schools in exchange for expansion of enrollments and revamping of curricula. Medicare legislation was enacted in 1965, thus expanding the access of a large portion of our population to medical services, and providing the funds to pay for these services.

To quote Cooper:

> These programs reflected a shift in the public demand and placed new pressures on the academic medical centers; more health care was required and more physicians were needed to provide it. [5]

He goes on to note that this development put further stress on the financial stability of the medical centers. By the late 1960s more than half of the medical schools in the United States were receiving assistance for financial distress. Cooper notes that the report of the Carnegie Commission in 1970 paid particular attention to the proposal to shorten the number of years in medical school from four to three. [6] A second issue raised in that report must not be overlooked: the emphasis on preparation of a less scientifically prepared physician, who would be able to treat common and simple emotional and organic problems, rather than a scholarly physician who dealt in great depth with illness. [7]

The *apparent* national commitment to support medical education which evolved in the early 1960s was expressed in legislation in the late 1960s. It provided the financial base for the expansion of enrollments and the modification of the curriculum. A host of reports on medical manpower and education during the last fifteen years have reinforced this avowal of national purpose and the federal funding that followed. The health professions schools of the United States were stated to be a national resource. Thus they would, and should, receive some support from federal sources, rather than be wholly dependent on funding from state government and private resources. The University of Nebraska College of Medicine and its other health professions schools responded by expanding enrollments and shortening the time between admission and award of the professional degree.

For those interested in a more detailed analysis of this "national mission" for the health professions, an unusually fine Ph.D. dissertation was written in 1968 by Roger L. Amidon: *Medical Education in the United States: A Nation's Call to Serve*.[8] In it he discusses the growing national emphasis on medical education and medical service.

A moment's reflection on these developments brings home the point that our national commitment to medical education and to national health insurance, as described in the middle 1960s and early 1970s, has not yet solidified and materialized. Who cannot recall in each recent year having heard the statement, "Certainly we will not have federal health insurance in the next twelve months, but undoubtedly within the year that follows a national health insurance program will be enacted by Congress." This prediction has yet to be realized, and with each day that passes there seems to be greater doubt about the outcome. The developments in medical education may well have received an impetus that pushed the medical schools beyond the national commitment, if federal legislation, or the absence of it, is in fact an accurate reflection of that intent.

The legislation of the mid-1960s, which focused on expansion of health services and *research in application of health services,* cited the university medical centers as the apparent natural resource. Lowell T. Coggeshall enunciated the philosophy that was developing in 1965:

> Clearly, past trends and implementation of the prevailing philosophy are expanding the role of government in the health care field as well as in the sponsorship of research and education. Expansion of the government's role is the logical consequence of a generally enlarged sense of public responsibility for national and individual health.[9]

This was the marching song of the 1960s. It led us to the stage at which we are today, and served as the philosophical background for the development of the three-year educational program at the University of Nebraska College of Medicine.

It must be noted parenthetically that during World War II several medical schools in the United States introduced a three-year educational program in response to an unusual national need. In general they simply accelerated the rate at which students proceeded through the curricula of those schools. It seems appalling that, with our current concern about evaluation of educational programs, we find no publications that assess the results of those modified curricula. The publications that have been available to us simply stated a few opinions and subjective conclusions that were not substantiated by any objective criteria or data.[10, 11] To add to that subjectivity, it is virtually impossible today to distinguish those physicians who completed the wartime accelerated curricula from those who either preceded or succeeded them in the traditional four-year course.

The background for the introduction of the *twelve-quarter curriculum,* as we prefer to call it at the University of Nebraska, was described by Dean Rigby as follows:

In July, 1972, the University of Nebraska College of Medicine started its first full class of medical students in a 12-quarter curriculum.

The rationale for the new curriculum is that the faculty of the University of Nebraska College of Medicine, like other medical educators throughout the nation, are concerned about adapting medical education to the needs of new and different times. There is an awareness of the need to improve the quality of educational experiences and conduct this process in a shorter period of time.

An important consideration is the fact that many students are better prepared for medical school today than in the past. Additionally, the emphasis in medical education is changing from "knowing the facts" to knowing how to acquire, correlate, and apply information. Since there is an undeniable information explosion, the student must learn proportionately fewer facts and [have] more educational flexibility. Finally, medical school graduates [must] continue their education proportionately longer now.

The specific goals for the educational program in the twelve-quarter curriculum at Nebraska were defined as follows:

1. To create an environment for learning which will:
   a) Conserve the students' background and ability;
   b) Favor the development of the potential in each student;
   c) Nurture the skills of and desire for self-learning;
   d) Display the knowledge, skills, attitudes, values, and ethical principles upon which a gratifying professional career is built;
   e) Make each student analytical and constructively critical of what he observes—sees, hears, and reads;

   f) Inculcate in each student the determination to extend con-
      scientious care to patients, employing scientific and clinical
      excellence complemented by sympathetic understanding;
   g) Develop awareness of the resources in health, welfare, and
      education extant within a community with which the physician
      cooperates to bring optimal care to his patient; and
   h) Foster an understanding of the responsibilities of a physician
      to the individual patient and to the community, bearing in mind
      the social and economic climate in which medical care is given.
2. To evolve and refine a curriculum which:
   a) Is a coordinated whole;
   b) Presents an orderly progression of pertinent knowledge and
      skills;
   c) Reflects the interdependence of biological, behavioral, and
      clinical sciences; and
   d) Recognizes and permits advantage to be taken of the variations
      in backgrounds, interests, and career aims of individual stu-
      dents.
3. To monitor and evaluate the output of the curriculum by the best
   methods available, and to analyze the performance results in terms
   of the professed philosophy and goals of the faculty.
4. To involve students in the planning, conduct, and evaluation of
   the curriculum.
5. To seek, develop, and employ innovative approaches to course design, to teaching methods, and to evaluative procedures.
6. To organize teaching functions of each department or discipline in
   a manner that protects scholarly pursuit and research and permits
   graduate educational programs to flourish.

Table 1 illustrates the twelve-quarter curriculum at the University
of Nebraska College of Medicine. The faculty devised three phases
in the curriculum composed of twelve blocks of twelve weeks each.
The first four-quarter phase consists essentially of introduction to
the basic medical sciences, although it does include introduction
to clinical medicine. Phase II, the transition phase, has two quarters,
dominated by introduction to and correlation of clinical concepts.
Phase III consists of clinical rotations made up of six periods for
clerkships on a varied rotational basis. Traditional clerkships in
medicine, surgery, psychiatry, obstetrics and gynecology, and pediatrics are each of eight weeks' duration. Family practice preceptorships, and ambulatory medicine and neurosciences are each
four-week required clerkships. Electives are available for four- to
twelve-week periods.

Analysis of the first six quarters reveals a heavily scheduled period in which all students are subjected to the same courses. The seventh through the twelfth quarters are composed of four-week divisions, which permit greater flexibility in the arrangement of clerkships.

In considering the advantages and disadvantages of the twelve-quarter curriculum in a three-year program as provided by the university, we find several simple and subjective observations that may be labeled as *advantages:*

1. Completion of the M.D. course in three years offers the opportunity for a physician to be available as an independent practitioner for one more year in his total career.

2. Since the program permits a student to complete the requirements for the M.D. degree in one less year, living costs are therefore reduced by a year.

3. A three-year program permits concentrated learning with shorter intervals of time away from the newly acquired knowledge before it is applied at the next level of responsibility in medicine. Some may consider this a disadvantage.

4. Three-year curricula have tended to reduce the time allocated to traditional basic science presentations in basic science departmental programs. This training is often relocated in the clinical clerkships, or in educational courses presented by clinical departments.

5. The mere introduction of change in the curriculum has stimulated both faculty and students to devote more attention to the educational program itself. The result may well be improved education, at least during the first few years following the change, merely by virtue of the change.

6. The twelve-quarter curriculum at Nebraska provides flexibility in educational opportunities for students, including the possibility of extending the curriculum over four calendar years to fit a student's secondary educational needs or goals.

7. The faculty has reviewed the curriculum to reduce redundancies in teaching, and has a better understanding of the educational goals of the curriculum as they have defined them.

These are the *disadvantages* of our twelve-quarter curriculum:

1. The student may be one year younger at the time he receives his M.D. degree. This raises the question: Is he less mature than graduates of a four-year curriculum?

2. The shortened program may tend to encourage students who

TABLE 1. TWELVE-QUARTER CURRICULUM, UNIVERSITY OF NEBRASKA COLLEGE OF MEDICINE, 1974–75

Phase I

(1)		(2)		(3)		(4)	
Biochemistry	96	Biochemistry	16	Physiology	102	Microbiology	84
Anatomy (gross, histology, neuro-anatomy, embroyology)	190	Anatomy (gross, histology, embryology)	136	Microbiology	84	Pathology	84
Clinical medicine	78	Physiology	101	Pathology	84	Pharmacology	48
Human ecology	12	Pharmacology	12	Pharmacology	24	Basic psychiatry	36
	376	Clinical medicine	92	Clinical medicine	96	Epidemiology	12
Unscheduled	152	Human ecology	12	Human ecology	12	Clinical medicine	96
	528		369		402		360
		Unscheduled	159	Unscheduled	126	Unscheduled	168
			528		528		528

Phase II (Transition)

(5)		(6)	
Vacation: 5 weeks		Clinical pathology	84
Ophthalmology	21	Clinical pharmacology	18
Pathology	12	Mechanisms of disease	56
Genetics	18	Cardiovascular	20
Pharmacology	24	Reproductive medicine	40
Review		Dermatology	18
Radiology	8	Matrix	120
Medical jurisprudence	12		356
Life support	10	Unscheduled	172
Problems in medicine	20		528
Hematology	8		
	133		
Unscheduled	395		
	528		

Phase III (Clinical Rotations)

(7)		(8)	
Medicine clerkship	8 weeks	Surgery clerkship	
Surgery clerkship	8 weeks	Psychiatry clerkship	
		(Continued 8 weeks from previous quarter)	

(Clerkship Sequence Random—Not Fixed)

(9)	(10)	(11)	(12)
Elective Obstetrics/ Gynecology Clerkship	Obstetrics/ Gynecology Clerkship Pediatrics Clerkship	Community preceptorship Out-patient medicine Elective	Elective Neuro-science
4 weeks 4 weeks 8 weeks	(Continued 8 weeks from previous quarter)	4 weeks 4 weeks 4 weeks	4 weeks 4 weeks
			(Optional vacation in place of one elective)

Graduation May

perform well to maintain the pace, but they may not take advantage of opportunities to extend the educational program. Extension may be interpreted by classmates as being an attempt on the part of the individual student or the faculty to assist the student to compensate for unsatisfactory performance.

3. There is a critical dependence on graduate medical education—house officeships, internships, and residencies—for adequate preparation of the physician for practice. This is a disadvantage, because the responsibility for this important phase of education now shifts to the student and away from the university.

4. The students must make decisions about graduate medical education and future career choices before they have completed rotations in the required clerkships. These clerkships are not only essential to the students in their principal educational program, but important factors in influencing their decisions on medical practice.

5. There may be too great a tendency to reduce time devoted to the basic sciences of medicine. Thus students may enter the clinical years with basic science information that is too shallow for them to reap the greatest educational benefit, particularly for the earlier clerkships.

6. Students in the accelerated twelve-quarter curriculum have less free time away from school, and thus have reduced opportunities for employment to help finance the costs of attending medical school.

7. There is some stigma attached to extending the twelve-quarter curriculum over a four-year period, but it varies with succeeding classes. At Nebraska there was an initial sense of esprit de corps, and all students sought to complete the twelve-quarter curriculum in three years without extension because they felt that was their commitment. In the next phase, the students who extended their educational programs were those who were having academic difficulty. We are now seeing a third phase, in which the superior student is choosing to extend, and is doing so without apology.

8. Students do experience a pressure of time if they are not provided the opportunity for a vacation or some break in their educational program.

9. If the three-year and the four-year students are considered as two separate classes, a strong interclass hostility may arise.

But what about more objective information on advantages and disadvantages of the shortened educational programs?

Studies of the University of Nebraska's medical students indicate that the average age of those in the twelve-quarter curriculum and those in the last class to finish under the four-year curriculum in May 1975 was virtually identical at the time of their admission to medical school (Table 2). The average age *on admission* of the twelve-quarter group of 123 students graduating in 1975 was twenty-three; the average age *on admission* of the four-year class of ninety-seven students graduating in May 1975 was also twenty-three. When they entered medical school, the scores for both groups on the Medical College Admission Test (MCAT) were similar, and not significantly different by statistical evaluation (Table 3). The mean science scores were 550.27 for students entering the twelve-quarter curriculum, and 545.81 for the four-year students. The mean scores on the quantitative tests were 593.40 and 609.80, respectively.

As the students proceeded through the curricula they took the only nationally standardized examinations available to medical schools: Parts I and II of the National Board of Medical Examiners (NBME). Again, tabulation of these data shows no great variation in the performance of these two groups of students (Table 4). The mean total scores on Part I were 500.87 for the twelve-quarter students, and 508.40 for the four-year students. The difference in the two values is not significant by the *t* test. Part II mean total scores were 473.28 and 476.60, again showing no important variation (Table 5).

Graduate students now seeking appointments as house officers are having difficulties because of changes in the graduate medical educational programs. The elimination of the rotating internship, which is not related to the residency, has frustrated some students. As a consequence many have chosen to enter family practice residency programs in order to gain a broader medical information base. These students may later opt to enter another of the specialty

TABLE 2. AGE COMPARISON ON BEGINNING UNDERGRADUATE MEDICAL EDUCATION: TWELVE-QUARTER AND FOUR-YEAR CLASSES GRADUATING MAY 1975, UNIVERSITY OF NEBRASKA COLLEGE OF MEDICINE

Class	Age Range	Mean	Standard Deviation
Twelve-quarter	20 yrs. 0 mos.-36 yrs, 0 mos.	23.37 yrs.	2.43
Four-year	20 yrs. 8 mos.-31 yrs. 8 mos.	23.12 yrs.	2.00

$t = .0789$. Difference between groups is nonsignificant. A critical t value of ± 1.98 is required for significance.

TABLE 3. MEDICAL COLLEGE ADMISSION TEST SCORES TWELVE-QUARTER AND FOUR-YEAR STUDENTS GRADUATING MAY 1975, UNIVERSITY OF NEBRASKA COLLEGE OF MEDICINE

Class	Verbal		Quantitative		General Information		Science	
	Mean	S.D.	Mean	S.D.	Mean	S.D.	Mean	S.D.
Twelve-quarter	523.09	79.72	593.40	76.66	519.85	71.85	550.27	76.18
Four-year	530.82	81.09	609.80	62.42	537.35	68.72	545.81	57.72
	$t=.7201$		$t=1.7433$		$t=1.8604$		$t=.4862$	

Differences between groups on all subtests were nonsignificant. A critical t value of ± 1.98 is required for significance.

TABLE 4. NATIONAL BOARD OF MEDICAL EXAMINERS PART I
EXAMINATION IN THE BASIC MEDICAL SCIENCES (TOTAL SCORES):
TWELVE-QUARTER AND FOUR-YEAR CLASSES GRADUATING MAY 1975
UNIVERSITY OF NEBRASKA COLLEGE OF MEDICINE

Class	Mean Score	Standard Deviation
Twelve-quarter	500.87	71.43
Four-year	508.40	76.67

$t = .7641$. Difference between groups is nonsignificant. Critical t value for significance is ± 1.98.

areas, however, instead of proceeding into the second and third years of the family practice residency. Reintroduction of the flexible year of graduate education may be a very important response to these special needs of students as they finish undergraduate medical education.

Medical schools in the United States are faced not only with the advantages and disadvantages of the shortened curriculum as described here, but with the realities of responding to the apparent intent and desire to solve what has been labeled as a national crisis in the shortage of health professionals. The medical schools now find themselves in a situation where they have assumed a massive undertaking to expand enrollments and revise curricula— steps that place great demands on faculty. Commitment to this national goal must obviously be questioned, however, in view of current federal legislative and administrative actions. Certainly there are pressures to reduce the tax burden on individuals and to shift tax funds to support other major social purposes. But the disenchantment of the American medical schools with the fickle nature of a major commitment that lasts no longer than ten years, such as occurred from 1965 to 1975, will certainly be a reminder to others in this country who undertake a congressionally sponsored "national commitment."

TABLE 5. NATIONAL BOARD OF MEDICAL EXAMINERS PART II
EXAMINATION IN THE CLINICAL SCIENCES (TOTAL SCORES): TWELVE-
QUARTER AND FOUR-YEAR CLASSES GRADUATING MAY 1975
UNIVERSITY OF NEBRASKA COLLEGE OF MEDICINE

Class	Mean Score	Standard Deviation
Twelve-quarter	473.28	78.60
Four-year	476.60	84.73

$t = .28$. Difference between groups is nonsignificant. Critical t value for significance is ± 1.98.

Public debate on such important national issues will certainly rage on, but meanwhile, without federal funds for education, the medical schools may be in worse financial straits in 1975 than they were a decade ago. Today the schools are finding a reduction in and termination of federal support for programs they have undertaken. They must seek to replace these funds from local government or private sources, which are being severely pressed to cope with other social issues. Alternatively, the schools may have to exist with reduced funds, either due to public reaction against increased local taxation or to apparent public antipathy toward the use of philanthropies as a route by which private monies are channeled to respond to public purposes.

To say that the medical schools and the other health education schools in the universities of the United States are facing a dilemma is an understatement. Uncertainty of continued funding for expanded and year-round teaching schedules must be a disadvantage to an institution adopting a shortened curriculum.

For the future, the University of Nebraska College of Medicine will solidify its financial support and stabilize the changes that have been made in the twelve-quarter curriculum. I would emphasize that while this curriculum is very similar to the former four-year program, it is available over a flexible period of time, the minimum being three years. This variability in the duration of medical education will probably receive continued support as more students take advantage of flexibility in the pace at which they may progress. More faculty members may see the attributes of having medical curricula offered on a twelve-month basis, in order to better balance the student load and match it with the other educational duties and institutional demands on their time for administrative and scholarly activities, in addition to their patient care responsibilities. The flexibility of the curriculum may well be the greatest advantage of a three-year educational program for the medical student, the faculty, and the administration and board of the university.

It is likely that in the nineteen schools that have now established a three-year medical educational plan the advantages will outweigh the disadvantages for both faculty and students and will serve the public well. The experience at the University of Tennessee, for example, where a three-year program has been in effect for many years, seems to support the likelihood that future medical education in those schools with three-year curricula will be solidified around such programs.

Those schools that wish to introduce an undergraduate medical curriculum offered over a three-year span should carefully weigh its advantages and disadvantages, based on their local circumstances. Certainly the only objective detectable advantage for the public is that one year of availability as a health professional has been added to the career of a physician. With the current move to expand economic incentives for earlier retirement, there may be great need to gain this one year. Certainly advancement of the retirement age of physicians from seventy to sixty-two years of age could have a profound impact on the reduction in the number of physicians practicing medicine, particularly in the midwestern United States.

A final evaluation of Nebraska's twelve-quarter curriculum must focus on the performance of the graduates as physicians. Small groups of students finished an accelerated program in 1973 and 1974, but neither these groups, nor the 1975 graduates, have been practicing long enough to permit valid observations. One of our goals is to define methods to evaluate these graduates in their practices and follow them through their careers. The advantages and disadvantages described in this report pertain only to the groups as undergraduate medical students.

Notes

1. Anne E. Crowley, ed., "Medical Education in the United States, 1973–74," *Journal of the American Medical Association, suppl.* 231 (January 1975): 6–33.
2. Ibid.
3. Ibid.
4. John A. D. Cooper, "External Forces Influencing Medical Education" in *The Changing Medical Curriculum: Report of a Macy Conference,* ed. Vernon W. Lippard and Elizabeth F. Purcell (New York: Josiah Macy, Jr. Foundation, 1972): 1–9.
5. Ibid.
6. Ibid.
7. *Higher Education and the Nation's Health: Policies for Medical and Dental Education,* A Special Report and Recommendations by the Carnegie Commission on Higher Learning (New York: McGraw-Hill Book Co., October 1970).
8. Roger L. Amidon, *Medical Education in the United States: A Nation's Call to Serve,* Health Care Research Series No. 7 (Iowa City: University of Iowa, 1968).
9. Lowell T. Coggeshall, *Planning for Medical Progress through Education* (Illinois: Association of American Medical Colleges, 1965).

10. Victor Johnson, "Annual Report: Medical Education in the United States," *Journal of the American Medical Association* 125 (19 August 1944): 1112–15.
11. ———, "Annual Report: Medical Education in the United States," ibid., 129 (1 September 1945): 41–42.

DISCUSSION

If students choose the family practice option they lose the year they supposedly gained in the shortened curriculum.

An increasing number of schools are becoming disenchanted with the three-year curriculum, feeling that it has become congested, with too many examinations and not enough time for faculty research. An evaluation of the accelerated curriculum is underway at Nebraska. Thus far it would appear that there is no major difference between the three-year and four-year students, although a growing number of them are opting for four years. It is still too early to tell whether there is a difference in the career orientations of the two groups.

Independent Study Programs: The State of the Art

GREGORY L. TRZEBIATOWSKI

When medical education began in the 1960s to break out of the hypnosis of the post-Flexnerian era and start the agonizing process of self-evaluation of curricula and instructional methods, a number of innovative curricular arrangements ensued. The shift to a continuous three-year curriculum, the use of a body systems approach, first attempted at Western Reserve University twenty-five years ago, and the integration of clinical and basic sciences through the clinical case approach—all are being tried in a number of medical schools. A wide variety of instructional technologies have come into use. Prominent among them are instructional television, audiovisual materials, programmed instruction, and, most recently, computer-assisted instruction.

One of the innovative instructional approaches, independent study programs (ISPs), is the subject of the present discussion. ISPs have always existed in medical schools: every school has had a few maverick students who chose not to attend lectures and developed their own special strategy of preparing for their mastery examinations. A number of schools now offer ISPs as an organized component of their total curriculum, however, the most notable being the programs of the Ohio State University, and the universities of Illinois, Washington, and Wisconsin.

Do these examples constitute a trend in medical education, or are they simply spurious attempts at innovation? Will they fall prey to the statistical phenomenon of regression toward the mean—the traditional lecture-discussion model? To try to assess the seriousness of this trend, a brief questionnaire was developed and sent to 110 medical schools in the United States. Before discussing the results of the survey, I would like to attempt to define independent study,

111

to explore very briefly the educational rationale for it, and to summarize the developments in those medical schools that have major ISPs.

DEFINITION OF INDEPENDENT STUDY

There is no widely accepted definition of independent study. Paul Dressel of Michigan State University, one of the leading writers on higher education, offers this definition: "Independent Study is the student's self-directed pursuit of academic competence in as autonomous a manner as he is able to exercise at any particular time." [1] ISPs are, then, those academic programs that make it possible for the student to self-determine what he is to learn within parameters defined by the faculty; the rate at which he is to learn; and the mode of study or learning resources he is to use in mastering the objectives, in order to achieve a high level of subject matter mastery and to become a self-directed, lifelong learner.

Since independent study can take place anywhere along the didactic-independent study continuum, as shown in Table 1, for purposes of this discussion I have divided it into two categories.

The first is *independent study activities*. These are activities on the part of the student, either by his own volition or without direct supervision of the faculty. Going to the library to find and read a research paper on a topic to be covered in a future lecture, without being told to do so by a faculty member, is an example of independent study. Other examples are the student's use of programmed texts, computer-assisted instruction materials, slide-tape programs,

TABLE 1. THE DIDACTIC-INDEPENDENT STUDY CONTINUUM

Pure Didactic			*Pure ISP*
ISP Activities	Minor ISP		Major ISP
$\longleftarrow$			$\longrightarrow$
Faculty Controls:		Student Controls:	
Content presented		Program or project goals	
Objectives		Objectives to be	
Texts and other		mastered	
learning resources		Learning resources	
Laboratory exercises		used	
Tests		Study environment	
Rate of progress		Rate of progress	
Normative standards		Evaluation by contact	
		with faculty	

and video cassettes independent of a faculty member, although he may have been assigned specifically to work with these materials.

I have arbitrarily broken the second major category into two segments:

1. *Minor ISPs* encompass a curricular unit, usually a course. The criterion used for separating minor programs from activities is that a student is given a grade in recognition of his achievements on an independent basis; his total grade is earned as a result of such activities.

2. *Major ISPs* are very similar to minor programs, except they usually permit independent rates of progress through large segments of the curriculum, which can affect the student's time of graduation. He may graduate early, due to a faster rate of progress than the traditional program allows, at the normal time, or later, as a result of a slower pace or of having elected to enrich his curriculum with additional material that takes him longer to master.

Why would a medical school want to develop a program in which students appear to take control of their own education? Some obvious answers are: 1) to provide for the exceptional student who is bored by the pace set for the majority of the class; or 2) to provide a remedial, slow-paced program for the disadvantaged student who cannot keep up. While these are legitimate grounds for independent study, more significant reasons were alluded to in the definition, that is, a genuine interest in developing into a truly self-directed independent learner.

A hematologist friend remarked in a casual conversation that almost everything worth knowing about hematology had been discovered in the past five years, and that with the rate and size of malpractice suits one cannot afford not to keep up to date. We must prepare independent learners who are not afraid to assess themselves, determine their weaknesses, and set up a program to remedy them. The assumption is that an independent learner as a medical student will be an independent learner as a physician. This hypothesis remains to be tested.

Other reasons for shifting to ISPs have a much better research base and have been proven in practice. Educational psychologists point out that each of us develops our own individual learning style based on our personality and on our previous learning experiences.[2] Some learners are meadowlarks who learn more effectively early in the morning; others are owls who are most effective after midnight.

Some are print-oriented; some audio-oriented; while others need to do experiments and see it happen in order to completely grasp the material. Most important, as any teacher knows, each of us learns at a different rate. To further complicate the process, we learn different subject matter at different rates: we may learn material that is heavily mathematically oriented very slowly, and philosophical material very fast. Some can memorize lists, such as those of bones and muscles, very quickly; others have great difficulty.

All learners need feedback on demand. Not the forced feedback of the Skinner-type programmed instruction after each small step of learning, nor every six weeks after a midterm examination—it should be available when needed. Finally, every student will learn more, and more efficiently, if what is expected of him is clearly specified. A great deal of psychological energy is expended in trying to "psych out" the professor to determine what he expects. What will be asked on the mastery exam should never be a mystery. Educational psychologists also tell us that in order to maximize retention of newly learned material, it is essential that the student discuss it with professors and other students. The purpose of these discussions is to clarify, embellish, and refine the material, and to ingrain it into the student's logic structure.

Many of a student's individual idiosyncracies can be accommodated through an ISP; independent study students have some of the best attitudes toward learning of any group I have encountered. They do not seem to develop the intense dislike of the basic sciences one so often finds in medical students; they find out quickly, as a general principle, that learning takes place as a direct result of their own thinking and not as a result of the exterior pressures of faculty members who will soon pass from their lives.

BRIEF SUMMARY OF MAJOR INDEPENDENT STUDY PROGRAMS

Several medical schools have developed ISPs that can be considered major innovative efforts. The schools mentioned here were chosen primarily because each has adopted a different type of program: Ohio State uses a fixed body-systems curriculum; the University of Illinois James Scholar Program, an unstructured student-determined curriculum; and the University of Illinois School of Basic Medical Sciences in Urbana–Champaign, a clinical case approach. Two others, the universities of Washington and Wisconsin, have successfully adapted and improved the program of another school, in this case Ohio State. The author's familiarity with the programs was also a major factor in citing them here.

Ohio State University Program

Grant O. Graves, chairman of the Department of Anatomy, began experimenting with independent study in 1962. The first class in the 1962–63 school year was arbitrarily divided into two groups —the independent study track and the traditional lecture-laboratory track. The results of that first year's experiment taught two valuable lessons: first, that students could learn as well in an ISP as they could by traditional methods; second, that they should enter the experimental program voluntarily, since there were students in both tracks who wanted to be in the other.

After several more years of experimentation it became evident that feedback mechanisms were needed to provide students with self-assessment information in order for them to determine how effectively they were progressing. ISP students received some of the highest and, unfortunately, lowest scores in the class—many of those with low scores were shocked to learn they were doing so poorly. Each year several improvements were made in the program. Experimentation was begun in 1967, for example, using computer-assisted instruction to provide the student with self-evaluation quizzes, thus eliminating the surprises at final grade time. By 1969, 71 percent of the class was volunteering to take the independent study track and was learning anatomy as effectively or more effectively than in the traditional track.

This early demonstration gave the college the impetus to write a proposal to extend ISPs to all six basic science subjects and to begin experimenting with a much larger program. In July 1969 the proposal was funded for three years by the then Bureau of Health Manpower. A small staff of six basic scientists, one from each department, eight part-time clinicians, a project director, and a medical educator conceptualized the program and drew up a curriculum to run from July 1969 to July 1970. The first class of thirty-two students was admitted into the ISP on an experimental basis. Two control groups were identified in the lecture-discussion track—one consisted of thirty-two students who volunteered to enroll in the ISP, but were not selected, and thirty-two who had not volunteered, but who had similar capabilities to those who entered the program.

That was a very hectic July, since the college had decided a year earlier to convert to a three-year, body systems curriculum for all students as of July 1970. The decision to adopt a three-year course is still hotly debated because the two faculty study groups that were a part of the year-long seminar on medical education came up with opposite findings: one proposed a return to a four-year curriculum with a three-year option; the other recommended staying with the three-year course and having a four-year option. It is of interest that student performance in the three-year curriculum was not a factor in the issue.

The major ISP features that were identified in 1969 still remain its chief characteristics, as follows:

1. Well-defined objectives are specified for the entire basic science curriculum (Figure 1). These are grouped into modules corresponding to body systems and broken into two major sequences: normal body systems and pathophysiology. Although not planned, the ISP curriculum parallels the fifteen-month lecture-discussion track program.

2. Learning resources, either purchased or developed, were tied directly to each of the objectives. These resources are used on a cafeteria basis by the students, depending on their personal preferences.

3. Each student passes through the modules at an independent rate. The most rapid progress to date was ten months. Maximum time to complete the basic sciences has been set at twenty-two months. A student may enter the twenty month clinical portion of his curriculum at the beginning of any month. Independent order of movement through the modules was tried the first year, but abandoned because it was not being used by the students, and it was too difficult to make each module free-standing.

4. Formative evaluation is provided through a computer-based tutorial evaluation system (TES) that also serves as the basis of the computer-based management system. Each student spends approximately one to one and one-half hours a week on the computer.

5. A total of seven mastery quizzes are taken by the students after they have passed through several modules. A shelf copy of the national board, utilizing only the biochemistry, physiology, and anatomy sections, is used at the end of the course on normal man. The passing of Part I of the national board examinations and satisfactory performance on a combined essay-oral test are the final requirements.

6. Faculty members serve primarily as tutors and advisors. The only planned group presentations are the clinical correlation sessions.

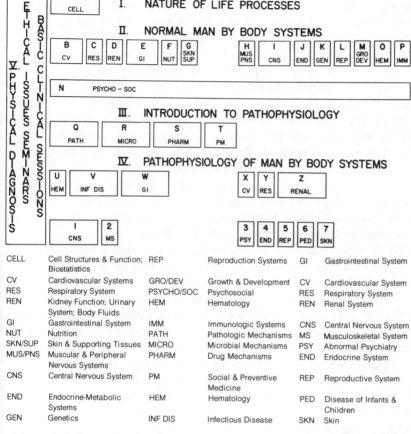

CELL   Cell Structures & Function;   REP   Reproduction Systems   GI   Gastrointestinal System
     Biostatistics
CV   Cardiovascular Systems   GRO/DEV   Growth & Development   CV   Cardiovascular System
RES   Respiratory System   PSYCHO/SOC   Psychosocial   RES   Respiratory System
REN   Kidney Function; Urinary   HEM   Hematology   REN   Renal System
     System; Body Fluids
GI   Gastrointestinal System   IMM   Immunologic Systems   CNS   Central Nervous System
NUT   Nutrition   PATH   Pathologic Mechanisms   MS   Musculoskeletal System
SKN/SUP   Skin & Supporting Tissues   MICRO   Microbial Mechanisms   PSY   Abnormal Psychiatry
MUS/PNS   Muscular & Peripheral   PHARM   Drug Mechanisms   END   Endocrine System
     Nervous Systems
CNS   Central Nervous System   PM   Social & Preventive   REP   Reproductive System
     Medicine
END   Endocrine-Metabolic   HEM   Hematology   PED   Disease of Infants &
     Systems   Children
GEN   Genetics   INF DIS   Infectious Disease   SKN   Skin

Figure 1. Independent Study Program Curriculum, Ohio State University.

Source: Elizabeth S. Ruppert and Robert Folk, "The Pediatric Role in the Independent Study Program," *Journal of Medical Education* 49, no. 11 (1974): 1064–66.

Faculty Role. The ISP is staffed by basic scientists and clinicians who function chiefly as tutors. Clinicians provide small-group correlation sessions to give the students an opportunity to become familiar with the vocabulary and to begin thinking clinically very early in their training. Faculty members perform anatomy prosections and provide microbiology and pathology laboratory experiences as small groups of students reach that stage of their studies. When the program was in its third year of operation, faculty members averaged four hours a week in active one-on-one tutoring with students, and another hour in revision of material. The remainder of the students' time is free for research and other activities. One of the disadvantages is that when the bolus of students in a class are passing through a particular module, some faculty members spend almost full-time in tutoring; this drops off to zero time later in the year.

The TES computer-based questions are written by the faculty for each module in the curriculum. The questions provide the student with feedback for both correct and incorrect answers. Although the TES questions can do much of the tutoring, faculty members, using the students' responses on the printout as a guide, do "fine grain" tutoring in a one-on-one tutorial session.

Faculty members are happy with the ISP, since it gives them very personal contact with students over an extended period of time. Their major objections are to rewriting the objectives and to preparing learning resources and the computer-based TES questions. The TES provides the basis for the management system that gives the program director a printout of each student's rate of progress and a variety of other managerial information.

Program Effectiveness. Employing a combination of hard and soft data to evaluate the ISP's effectiveness, after five years of careful scrutiny it can be concluded that it is more effective than the traditional lecture system. Expansion of the program has been delayed due to a shortage of faculty in the college, since increases in the enrollment were not accompanied by a commensurate increase in the size of the faculty. The college plans to raise the number of places in the ISP in July 1976 to approximately one hundred students out of the class of 227.

Using student satisfaction as a criterion, our medical students have been the best recruiters of others to the ISP. Its capability to accommodate individual needs, especially in terms of rates of progress, has been greatly appreciated by the students. Using the national boards as a "hard" criterion, the ISP is significantly more effective when compared to a matched group of students from the lecture-discussion phase curriculum. Three groups of medical educators who served as external auditors were invited in for a three-day visit, and each group's report clearly indicated that after examining a number of its facets the ISP is in their judgment a success.

The ISP has been less effective with minority and other disadvantaged students, since its materials were not especially written with those groups in mind. They seem to need a more structured environment than the ISP provides. A major hurdle for disadvantaged students is the requirement that they pass Part I of the national boards as a candidate. In addition to the ISP and the lecture-discussion program, a third track called the "Individualized Program" has been developed for disadvantaged students.[3]

Given the high correlation between performance on Parts I and II of the national boards, independent study students maintain their superiority over the lecture-discussion students when they take Part II of the boards at the time of graduation. A subjective evaluation of clinical performance, using the college's Clinical Evaluation Form, shows no significant differences between the two groups. Plans are being made to follow the students into their internships and residencies, and, if possible, into practice.

The University of Washington Program (WISP)[4]

Faculty at the University of Washington School of Medicine decided in 1971 to develop an ISP for their undergraduate curriculum. Subsequent to a visit to the Ohio State ISP in June 1972, the decision was made to adopt a similar program in time for the fall quarter. Computerized materials were made available via the Lister Hill National Center for Biomedical Communications. Under the direction of Ralph Cutler of the Clinical Research Center, a faculty was appointed and modification of the Ohio State program began.

Given the extremely short length of time between the decision to adopt the ISP and enrollment of the first class of twenty students, changes were made immediately to bring the materials into closer line with the existing University of Washington curricular objectives. While problems arose in the first year because of the haste with which the ISP was put into operation, student enthusiasm and dedication to the program remained high. It has followed the basic outlines of the Ohio State program, but one major difference is in the way faculty members are used. At Ohio State a defined faculty is assigned to the ISP, whereas at Washington it was decided to make departments responsible for student tutoring and the revision and updating of the ISP materials.

Although the transplantation process was not without difficulties, it has been judged a success.[5] Forty-three medical students are currently enrolled in WISP, including students from the WAMI program, an innovative effort described by Roy Schwartz in another chapter of this volume. While it is still too early to draw definite conclusions as to the effectiveness of the program, preliminary data comparing national board scores suggest that WISP students' performance is equivalent and possibly superior to that of lecture-discussion students. Students and faculty seem to appreciate the program's flexibility, as evidenced by the popularity of its use in Ph.D.–M.D programs and the WAMI program.

The University of Wisconsin [7]

The University of Wisconsin Medical School has developed an ISP based, in general, on the Ohio State model, but, like the University of Washington, it has made a number of valuable adaptations. Wisconsin's ISP, like Ohio State's, serves as an alternate method of study for the two-year basic science portion of the curriculum for up to thirty volunteer students a year. It provides: 1) clearly stated learning objectives; 2) self-paced, multiple learning paths; 3) an orientation program to enable the students to understand how the faculty is going to determine they have attained the objectives; 4) a special program to help students understand their own personal learning styles; 5) opportunities for frequent self-assessment to monitor progress; and 6) opportunities to interact with faculty as student need arises.

Program Differences. The faculty at the University of Wisconsin has developed a discipline-oriented curriculum that is compatible with the regular traditional curriculum. For example, some courses in the ISP, such as physiological chemistry, are controlled by the traditional program, presumably because ISP students and regular curriculum students are scheduled into the same laboratories. Another major difference is that self-assessment examinations are not computer-based, but serve essentially the same function. The ISP curriculum is divided into two phases corresponding to the traditional first and second years. Courses are grouped by level within each phase, and students may progress through the courses within a group in any order they choose, thus offering them multiple learning paths. The ISP has not been operational long enough to determine its long-term effectiveness. Plans are being developed to follow up the program's graduates.

The University of Illinois James Scholar Program [8]

This ISP is unique in that the student is treated as an honor student, in much the same way as an undergraduate baccalaureate honor student is treated. A James scholar is given tremendous freedom to determine the curriculum he studies. In this respect, of all the ISPs currently in operation the James Scholar Program is the closest to a pure independent study program.

Historical Background. In 1967 the University of Illinois College of Medicine identified the need to develop a program that would produce a self-reliant and self-directed learner. The ISP was established to provide a small group of highly motivated students, judged to have the capacity to do independent, creative work, with the knowledge and means to progress through medical school at their own pace, thereby encouraging and reinforcing individual styles.

Student Selection. The selection of students for the ISP is based on applications received from interested freshmen and on subsequent individual and group interviews. About forty students, or 20 percent, of the freshmen class respond to an invitation to join the ISP. After the interviews some students elect to withdraw from consideration; of the remaining group, twenty are enrolled in the program as their means of acquiring the M.D. degree.

Program Requirements. Students in the ISP are still subject to the academic requirements of the College of Medicine. In order to qualify for the M.D. degree, they must pass the same certifying examinations required of all medical students, successfully complete an in-depth study, and demonstrate an acceptable degree of clinical problem-solving ability as determined by supervising faculty. Students in the ISP are not required to complete a certain number or kind of clinical clerkships. Most students elect the five major clinical clerkships, however—medicine, pediatrics, obstetrics and gynecology, surgery, and psychiatry—as well as a variety of subspecialty clinical experiences.

The Program. The James scholar ISP is unique in that each student plans, implements, and evaluates his academic activities in consultation with a faculty advisor. In addition, students have the services of a departmental counselor from each discipline who has been assigned this responsibility. Counselors help students identify basic concepts of the particular discipline, and direct them to educational resources that facilitate their study of that area. A wide variety of audiovisual materials are available for acquisition of the new knowledge and for self-testing during clinical studies. A student may, for example, practice clinical diagnostic skills by using models and various simulation equipment.

Program Impact. Although there are limited data at this time, the traditional academic achievements of ISP students do not appear to differ from those of students in the regular curriculum. This preliminary observation has been based on the absence of any statistically significant differences in scores between the two groups on Part I of the national boards. ISP students participate in a much wider variety of activities during medical school, however, and express a stronger interest to go into academic or scientific work after they have obtained their degrees.

University of Illinois College of Medicine, School of Basic Medical Sciences in Urbana–Champaign [9]

The School of Basic Medical Sciences in Urbana–Champaign began its first year of operation in 1972 with an ISP called "A One-Year Independent Study Experimental Approach." This ISP is unique in that it attempts to use classic clinical cases as its basis. All students enrolled at the school are admitted into an ISP that attempts to achieve two years of traditional studies in twelve months. The curriculum consists of eleven basic science disciplines, each broken down into independent learning units and ten classical clinical problems relating basic medical science to human disease.

The curriculum is divided into 300 units or learning packages, each developed in a standard format. Learning the basic science content units is accomplished in a guided study, problem-oriented mode using clinical problems. During the course of the first year the student is exposed to ten clinical problems to complete his coverage of the basic medical sciences, and acts as a beginning doctor in defining and understanding the basic science of each clinical problem. Patients are seen in the hospital, in the clinic, in the emergency room, or in a doctor's office. When the student encounters a basic science question relative to the clinical problem he is handling he turns to one of the 300 self-study units, which helps him master the basic science material needed to solve the problem.

A carefully worked out system of evaluation, starting with pretests and ending with oral examinations, assures that the student masters the material he is expected to learn. Extensive use is made of clinical faculty, both as M.D. preceptors and M.D. evaluators.

Program Evaluation. This ISP attempts to cover the content skills of the basic medical sciences in a single year. To this end, all sixteen of the students currently enrolled have successfully passed the University of Illinois's first-year comprehensive examination. Fifteen of the sixteen have passed the national boards, Part I. All are now enrolled in one of the three clinical schools of the university. The most striking aspects of this program are that, first, it requires all students enrolled in the school to participate in an ISP; second, the pacing of the program is very rapid; and third, a combination of discipline-oriented, self-learning units are integrated with clinical problems.

Results of the State-of-the-Art Survey

A brief questionnaire was mailed to 110 medical schools in the United States. The purpose of the survey was not to do a definitive study of ISPs in the schools, but to:

1. Determine which schools had ISPs and which did not, using the schools own definition of an independent study program;

2. Assess plans for future ISPs;

3. Determine the characteristics of present and future programs; and

4. Determine the major drawbacks to ISPs.

No definition of an ISP was offered, except that which could be inferred from the list of program characteristics. This was done to prevent putting undue restraints on the respondents. It is my feeling that ISPs are still in the developmental stage, and to operationally define independent study would eliminate some excellent programs. The University of Illinois James Scholar Program, for example, does not use objectives; most schools do. If objectives were a part of an operational definition, therefore, the James Scholar Program would not qualify. Independent study is more of a philosophical approach than a mechanistic technology such as programmed instruction.

Ninety-one of the 110 schools responded—an 83 percent return. Of the respondents, sixty, or 66 percent, indicated they did not now have an independent study course or program; thirty-one, or 34 percent, indicated they did have an ISP. This response compares with 58 percent positive responses reported by 135 medical schools, including Canadian schools, in the *1974–75 AAMC Curriculum Directory*.[10] The higher AAMC percentage may be due to the broader definition it used, which was that:

Independent Study refers to educational formats imposing neither specific course sequence nor prearranged time periods for student learning. Students develop their own learning programs but must satisfy faculty requirements.

Of the thirty-one schools with ISPs, eleven stated that they use them in the basic sciences only; seventeen schools had programs in both the basic science and clinical portions of their curricula. Of the ISPs currently operational, the survey showed that they are evenly distributed over all disciplines. As might be expected, the basic science programs are more structured than those in the clinical sciences. Current ISPs are organized under four formats: eighteen traditional; eight body systems; ten clinical cases; and two student-organized. Over one-half of the programs' students enter them voluntarily. Seventy-seven percent of the existing programs plan to expand their ISPs in the next two years.

The drawback to the programs are summarized below:

Schools with ISPs (Percent)		*Schools without ISP* (Percent)
49	High development cost	37
71	Shortage of interested faculty	58
7	Lack of administrative support	10
10	Lack of student interest	8
35	Complexity of program management	25
13	Questionable program effectiveness	27
26	More expensive than traditional	17
10	Other	5
10	No response	18

Several interesting factors should be noted in studying the drawbacks to the programs as perceived by those schools that have had experience with ISPs versus those that have not. The former recognize to a greater extent that gaining faculty interest is a major hindrance, and that the complexities of program management can be a drawback. On the other hand, schools that have ISPs do not question the programs' effectiveness nearly as much as those that do not have them.

Of the sixty schools without ISPs at the present time, 45 percent plan to develop one or more in the next two years. Almost all of these new programs will be in the basic sciences. There seems little question that, based on the survey data, ISPs are rapidly increasing in United States medical schools. Another telling factor is that over three-fourths of those schools that have ISPs plan to expand them.

CONCLUSIONS

The following conclusions are offered as a summary:

1. Independent study programs are at least as effective as traditional programs, and preliminary data indicate that in some schools they are more effective.

2. Students in ISPs have a much better attitude toward medical school, particularly toward their study of the basic sciences.

3. As a result of a national survey it can be concluded that there is a definite trend towards the development of ISPs in United States medical schools.

4. Independent study programs can serve a wide variety of purposes, including remedial, honors, and alternate track as a school's only program, as is the case at the University of Illinois School of Basic Medical Sciences in Urbana–Champaign.

5. Disadvantaged students need a special ISP, and work is needed in the development of such programs if this method of study is to be successfully used by these students.

6. Independent study programs and program models can be transplanted and successfully adapted by other medical schools.

7. A lack of faculty interest in developing and teaching in ISPs is a significant drawback.

8. The high cost of program development is perceived as a major problem. This cost can be decreased considerably by the adaptation of a program already in operation at another medical school.

9. The clinical case approach seems to offer more opportunities to apply basic science knowledge immediately than either the traditional disciplines or body-systems organization.

10. Long-term, follow-up studies need to be conducted to determine whether or not medical students who are trained in ISPs maintain their independent study skills throughout their professional careers.

Notes

1. Paul Dressel and Mary Thompson, *Independent Study* (San Francisco: Jossey-Bass Publishers, 1973): 1.

2. Robert Gagne, "Learning Research and Its Implications for Independent Learning," in *The Theory and Nature of Independent Learning,* ed. Gerald Gleason (Scranton, Pennsylvania: International Textbook Co., 1967): chap. 2.

3. Gregory Trzebiatowski, *Multitrack Instructional Systems for the Basic Sciences,* Paper presented at the Interdisciplinary Conference on Flexible

Education for the Health Professions in Iowa City, April 1975 (New York: John Wiley Jacobs Publishing Co., forthcoming).
4. Charles Dohner and N. F. Shannon, "A Description of the University of Washington Experience in Using the OSU ISP Curriculum, Part III—The Outcomes," in *Individualizing the Study of Medicine* (Oak Lawn, Illinois: Educational Products, Inc., forthcoming).
5. Ibid.
6. Ibid.
7. Howard Stone, "A Student Guide to the Independent Study Program at the University of Wisconsin–Madison School of Medicine," Report of the Independent Study Program at the University of Wisconsin (Undated monograph).
8. Charles Johns and Roger D. Smith, "An Independent Study Program in Medical School," *Journal of Medical Education* 48, no. 8 (1973): 732–36.
9. W. Sorlie et al., "Medical Basic Sciences—A One Year Independent Study Experimental Approach," Report of the University of Illinois College of Medicine (Undated monograph).
10. *1974–75 AAMC Curriculum Directory* (Washington: Association of American Medical Colleges, 1975).

DISCUSSION

Independent study programs (ISPs) are a problem for premedical students because many admissions committees have no faith in their preparation. Another participant took issue with this, saying that admissions committees look favorably on ISP applicants, providing sufficient documentation is given by the program director.

An ISP must operate within the parameters provided by the faculty, but it is important that students should participate in deciding on the objectives to be reached.

ISPs may be especially relevant for minority groups because the students can proceed at their own pace.

A major deterrant to adoption of ISPs is their expense.

The Elective Curriculum at Stanford University: Report on the First Three Graduating Classes

JOHN STEWARD * and CLAYTON RICH

Since 1968 the Stanford curriculum in medicine has been characterized by a very high degree of electivity and flexibility. Students generally have the option of selecting courses and clerkships they feel are appropriate in relation to their previous experience and to their career goals. The faculty accepts responsibility for the development of the courses and clerkships, subject to review and approval by departments and by the Committee on Courses and Curriculum. We shall report on the first three classes to graduate since this curriculum was introduced; describe the use of electives by students and faculty; and express our opinions on the current strengths and weaknesses of the program.

BACKGROUND

The major reason for moving the medical school from San Francisco to the Stanford University campus in Palo Alto in 1959 was to establish strong interactions in both education and research between the faculty in medicine and the faculty in other units of the university. The effects of this move on the school were profound. Not only were several additional, major basic science departments created, but, since many of the former faculty remained in San Francisco, the majority of the faculty in the clinical departments were new, young, and committed to the idea of becoming truly integrated with the intellectual life of the parent university.

The move brought the medical faculty to a campus that had

* Dr. Steward, associate dean, Stanford University School of Medicine, was not present at the conference.

already developed very extensive research programs in both the natural and social sciences and a strong commitment to graduate education. These themes continued in the following decade, fostered in part by federal support of research in biomedical and other areas of science. The emphasis on research, on the process of graduate education, and on a high degree of electivity for students became increasingly important throughout the university, including the medical school.

The first departure from a traditional medical curriculum occurred at the time of the move, when a mandatory five-year program was instituted. It consisted of three preclinical years followed by two clinical years. During the first three years, required basic science courses occupied approximately half of each day, the remaining time being available for the student to take elective courses in the medical school, or become involved in areas unrelated to medicine. This large amount of free time was valuable, particularly for students with strong research interests. Late in the first decade at Palo Alto, however, with increasing frequency students pressed for an earlier introduction to clinical work, and, because of financial constraints, expressed a wish to hasten their pace through medical school. Thus the five-year curriculum came to be seen by the faculty as too inflexible.

The current elective medical curriculum, inaugurated in the autumn of 1968, represented an attempt to retain, for those students who would take advantage of it, the electivity available in the five-year curriculum, while providing them with greater flexibility to alter the structure of their education as their interests and career goals changed.

THE ELECTIVE CURRICULUM

Several concepts were critical in the development of the elective curriculum. Most important by far was recognition of the enormous core of knowledge directly relevant to the understanding of health and disease and to the practice of medicine. This knowledge so far exceeds the amount an individual can possibly absorb that many important topics must be omitted from any curriculum that could be designed. Moreover, the rate of introduction of new knowledge and the resulting changes in practice are so great that no body of information acceptable in one year would be adequate five or ten years later.* Therefore, the curriculum had to be based on two concepts: that selectivity about what is to be taught is necessary; and that developing in the student-physicians the capacity to make selections on their own behalf is essential if they are to keep informed of current information during the decades of practice after graduation.

Stanford is fortunate in that it attracts exceedingly able students, who are intellectually mature and independent. It was not obvious to faculty or students that their ability to make choices and to take responsibility for their own proficiency as students and future physicians was less than, for example, graduate students in the sciences or humanities. Moreover, as part of the process of medical education, it was considered critical to instill a commitment to self-directed learning that is essential throughout a doctor's career. Finally, we had before us the model of graduate education in the sciences and humanities, involving as it does considerable individual responsibility and flexibility on the part of each student, who works with his thesis advisor toward exactly these goals of current technical competence and lifelong scholarly achievement.

For these reasons, and possibly others, our faculty decided against an attempt to define a core body of knowledge that every student would have to acquire; instead we attempted to create the learning environment of graduate students elsewhere in the university. The resulting curriculum, put into operation in 1968, may be described as follows.

Requirements for the medical degree at Stanford consist of:

1. Registration for a minimum of eleven academic quarters—thirty-three months—unless a student is given credit for appropriate work taken prior to matriculation in medical school, in which case the number of quarters cannot be less than nine.

2. Satisfactory completion of 192 academic units in courses approved by the Committee on Courses and Curriculum (CCC).

a) Sixty-four of these 192 units must represent clinical work;
b) Forty-eight of the sixty-four clinical units must come from clerkships in which the student carries a primary responsibility for the patient and is directly supervised by full-time faculty at Stanford or one of its major affiliated hospitals. The clerkships must include experience in three different departments.

---

* This is illustrated by the fact that approximately 50 percent of the questions on the examination administered by the American Board of Internal Medicine in 1970 would require different responses in 1975.

3. Satisfactory performance on Parts I and II examinations of the National Board of Medical Examiners (NBME). The student must, in addition, achieve a score on every subtest comparable to the overall passing score set by the NBME.

4. Demonstration of suitability for the practice of medicine, as evidenced by the assumption of responsibility for patient care and integrity in the conduct of clinical and research activities.

Thus in this curriculum the student has no required preclinical courses that must be taken and passed. Although three academic quarters of clinical clerkships are mandatory, including experiences in three different departments, no student *must* take, for example, a clerkship in pediatrics, surgery, psychiatry, or medicine. The balance between preclinical work and clinical clerkships is left to the student, within the constraints already expressed, as is the duration of his medical education.

There are several important constraints and adjuncts to this curriculum.

1. It is inherent in the concept of the curriculum that the faculty would have a commitment to the implications of electives. Thus not only would course offerings include the usual major areas of basic science and clinical education, but specialized and innovative teaching and counseling would be available.

2. The heavy emphasis on individualization brings an additional responsibility, in that the faculty must evaluate performance and suitability for practice on the basis of personal contacts, rather than rely mainly on results of examinations.

3. To achieve the maximum benefits from the curriculum, there would have to be an effective system of advising. Although several methods have been tried, this remains one of the most difficult aspects of the program.

4. Because not every student must, or does, take a course in every discipline usually considered essential for medical practice, it is by means of successful performance in a comprehensive examination that the faculty gains assurance of overall competence.

5. Finally, the Standing Committee on Student Performance, chaired by the dean, monitors and directs students who are in academic difficulty or whose suitability as future physicians is in question. Students come before this committee automatically whenever they achieve fewer than thirty-nine credits for satisfactory work in a year; accumulate more than nine units of unsatisfactory work in a year; or fail any subtest of Parts I or II of the national boards.

Further, students may be brought before the committee for any reason by the associate deans for student affairs. The committee can require additional or remedial work or additional examinations, dictate specific course and clerkship assignments, or temporarily or permanently remove a student from the school. Thus this committee may stipulate requirements above those that apply to all students, and these must be met before an M.D. degree is awarded.

Responsibility for the curriculum resides in the CCC, a school-wide committee with representation from the faculty-at-large rather than from departments—basic and clinical sciences faculty and several deans. It reports directly to the Faculty Senate. The charge to the CCC includes responsibility for: 1) defining the educational goals of the school, as well as their continuous evolution and innovation; certifying that graduates have met the criteria required for the M.D. degree; identifying a body of knowledge that all students must master; ensuring that curricular offerings adequately include those academic topics basic to the practice of medicine; and scheduling courses so they are available to most students.

EXPERIENCE WITH THE ELECTIVE CURRICULUM

How Has the Faculty Responded?

It was expected that there might be a proliferation of courses. A comparison of the three years—1966–67 (preelective curriculum), 1969–70 (second year of elective curriculum), and 1974–75 (seventh year of elective curriculum)—indicates there has been a small increase in the number of courses offered by our basic science departments, 10 percent more now than in 1966–67. On the other hand, the number of courses, excluding clinical clerkships, offered by the clinical departments has more than doubled, and the various clinical clerkships have increased by about 50 percent. These data probably reflect departmental strengths and balances peculiar to Stanford, and should not support a general conclusion.

Several comments may be made, however. The CCC had recommended that basic science material be offered in two sequences: one basic and concise, the other more detailed and advanced. This has not materialized. Excluding early clinical experiences, clerkships, individual study, seminars, research, clinics, etc., it is of interest to note that approximately 40 percent of course offerings represent individual faculty efforts that focus on the individual's area of special interest.

The number of hours of laboratory instruction offered annually had been falling for several years prior to 1966–67, when they totaled 825; they fell precipitously to about three hundred in 1969–70, and have remained at that level. This trend is not at all unique to Stanford, since many schools have seen a marked reduction in hours of laboratory instruction, but it is probable that in this case our curriculum has exaggerated the decrease. For many of our students the only "wet" laboratory course taken is medical microbiology; the other courses are essentially observational in nature.

For 1972–73 the faculty effort in the medical school was divided as follows: all instruction, including joint research and teaching and joint patient care and teaching, 44 percent; research, 34 percent; and patient care, 22 percent. In fourteen other medical schools, six public and eight private, comparable average figures are: all instruction, 45 percent; research, 28 percent; and patient care, 27 percent. Thus the balance of our faculty efforts among teaching, research, and patient care is comparable to that reported by other medical schools.

Another important phenomenon of medical faculty involvement at Stanford must also be described. On an entirely elective basis, reflecting a university-wide commitment to education, the faculty has been heavily engaged in educational programs in the university-at-large. In 1974–75, for example, 16 percent of all the faculty responsible for teaching freshman seminars to university undergraduates came from the medical school.

During 1973–74 our faculty undertook courses and clerkships for medical students representing 21,500 student-units (a five-unit course with 100 students equals 500 student-units); during the same period our faculty's instruction of students in schools of the university other than medicine was equated with 17,000 student-units. Although the total of student-units was close to equal, instruction outside the medical school obviously required far less effort, because the teaching was most frequently in the form of lectures for large undergraduate classes. Nevertheless, these figures confirm that the faculty of medicine has made substantial contributions to other parts of the university.

How Have Students Utilized the Options Available?

Three uses of electivity will be mentioned: total amount of time in medical school; omission of courses and clerkships that ordinarily would be part of a traditional curriculum; and evidence of special concentration in some field of academic work.

1. *Time in medical school.* The average number of total academic quarters of work toward the M.D. degree is remarkably constant for the three graduating classes—between thirteen and one-half and fourteen. If a student took four years to attain the degree, and had free only the summer between the first and second years, the number of academic quarters would amount to fourteen. We therefore conclude that the *average* duration of medical education at Stanford is not significantly different from that in many schools with traditional curricula. There is, however, a very substantial variation in the total number of quarters taken by individual students (Figure 1). The range varies from the required minimum of nine quarters to a maximum of twenty-two. Students taking more than fifteen quarters include those who participate in research or who have a special academic interest and some admitted with disadvantaged educational backgrounds. The average number of quarters of preclinical work for all students in the first three graduating classes was very close to seven.

The proportion of Stanford students graduating in three, four, five, or six calendar years is given in Table 1. Most of those graduating in three years had begun or completed graduate work in one of the basic medical sciences before matriculating in medical school. There was a significant drop in the number graduating in five years between the classes of 1973 and 1975. This may have been a response to the increased cost of medical education; the pressures

TABLE 1. DURATION IN CALENDAR YEARS OF MEDICAL EDUCATION AT STANFORD FOR 1973, 1974, AND 1975 M.D. RECIPIENTS

Duration in Calendar Years	Year M.D. Awarded		
	1973 92 M.D.'s (Percent)	1974 76 M.D.'s (Percent)	1975 81 M.D.'s (Percent)
3 years	1	5	7
4 years	37	51	51
5 years	59	44 (2 MSTP)*	38 (5 MSTP)*
6 years	3 (2 MSTP)*	0	4 (all MSTP)*

* Students participating in the Medical Scientist Training Program.

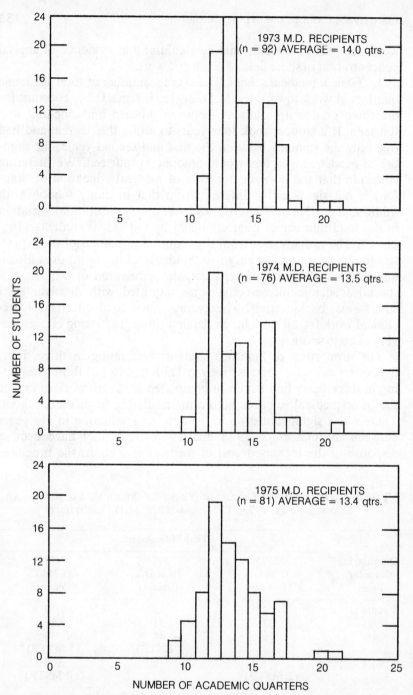

Figure 1. Total Number of Academic Quarters, Stanford University School of Medicine.

created by higher debts probably will continue to be responsible for fewer students electing a five-year program.

2. *Omission of courses and clerkships.* Table 2 shows the average percent of students in three graduating classes who formally took for credit basic sequences of courses in their preclinical curricula, as well as the average percent who formally took major basic clerkships. Many of our entering students had considerable exposure as undergraduates to disciplines such as biochemistry, genetics, and abnormal psychology. They often do not repeat these courses in medical school; others who have not taken introductory courses concentrate on advanced work in these areas or rely on self-study.

Although not required, all of our students take a clerkship in medicine. Over 90 percent of our graduates have also taken basic clerkships in surgery and pediatrics. Only three other clinical disciplines attract over 50 percent of our students: obstetrics and gynecology, radiology, and psychiatry.

Compared with the performance of the class as a whole, it is interesting to observe how students who did not participate in a basic science course performed on the national board subtest corresponding to the subject not taken. Twelve students who omitted one of the courses in 1973, and who had had prior work in the discipline, averaged at the 83rd percentile on those subtests (range

TABLE 2. FOR THE GRADUATING CLASSES OF 1973, 1974, AND 1975, THE AVERAGE PERCENTAGES OF M.D. RECIPIENTS FORMALLY COMPLETING MAJOR BASIC SCIENCE COURSE SEQUENCES AND BASIC CLINICAL CLERKSHIPS

Basic Course Sequences	Percent	Clinical Clerkships	Percent
Biochemistry (2 of 2 quarters)	77	Anesthesia	35
Gross anatomy	98	Dermatology	44
Histology	98	Community medicine	14
Neuroanatomy	97	Gynecology/obstetrics	79
Human genetics	41	Medicine	100
Clinical physiology			
(3 of 3 quarters)	94	Neurology	24
Pharmacology (2 of 3 quarters)	97	Pathology	41
Medical microbiology	89	Pediatrics	92
Pathology (2 of 2 courses)	85*	Psychiatry	60
Introduction to psychiatry	70	Radiology	73
Hematology	92	Surgery	96
Laboratory medicine	89	Emergency room	36
Physical diagnosis	98		

* For 1974 and 1975 graduating classes: 97 and 95 percent respectively.

65th to >99th), while eighteen who had had no prior formal instruction averaged at the 60th percentile (range 35th to >99th); the class as a whole averaged at the 78th percentile. Seven students in the three graduating classes who had not taken a surgical clerkship averaged at the 25th percentile (range 4th to 56th) in the surgery subtest of Part II of the national boards, and ten who did not take pediatrics clerkships averaged at the 34th percentile (range 7 to 90th). The classes as a whole were at the 57th and 74th percentile, respectively, in these two subtests.

3. *Use of other academic options.* The proximity of the Stanford Medical Center to the main quadrangle of the university facilitates course work by medical students in schools other than medicine. About 25 percent of our medical students take one or more courses elsewhere, and about 15 percent take three or more. In order of frequency, these courses are in music, a foreign language, anthropology, engineering, sociology, and psychology. An occasional student will receive an advanced degree in English or philosophy while in medical school.

Many students are attracted to Stanford because of an interest in research. Some may participate superficially for only a short while, but a substantial number—almost 25 percent for the 1975 graduating class—become sufficiently involved to author or coauthor scholarly publications. At any given time, between thirty and forty of our approximately three hundred and eighty medical students participate in the Medical Scientist Training Program, enrollment in which requires one year of full-time research and several other years of part-time research. Although these students are not encouraged to get the Ph.D. degree, a few do so.

Does the Elective Curriculum Adequately Prepare Students for the Practice of Medicine?

It is extremely difficult to determine the relationship between *any* curriculum and the effectiveness of its graduates in practice. We have no information on this point, and, in fact, we assume that the intelligence, judgment, personal involvement, and integrity of the student, not the content of the curriculum, determine his future performance. Indeed this assumption is fundamental to the concept of the elective curriculum.

Information exists that suggests our students perform exceedingly well, and that this capacity is not diminished as a result of their participation in the elective curriculum. The three graduating classes have held the same place (with a variation, up or down, of a few schools), when ranked against the student bodies of other schools nation-wide, with regard to both the MCAT and Parts I, II, and III of the national boards—the national ranking for the last of the three classes is not yet available for Parts II and III. These rankings have been remarkably consistent, neither significantly higher nor lower for the MCAT than for the national boards. In the past several years they have been slightly higher than before the introduction of the elective curriculum. Thus students who did well on examinations prior to admission to Stanford medical school continue to do well during and after participation in our elective curriculum.

On a systematic basis, William Creger, our associate dean for clinical student affairs, solicits evaluations from program directors on the performance of medical students in their first year of graduate medical education. The findings indicate they have had an increasingly good record in the past three years. We assume that the quality of our students and the growing emphasis on clinical medicine are among factors responsible for this.

Advantages of the Elective Curriculum

One can cite several advantages of a procedural nature, which are relatively apparent, and two others less easy to document, which at the same time are more important.

1. Students who have gained relevant knowledge in college or through special studies do not need to repeat such work in medical school.

2. Students with educational deficiencies can make them up at their own pace, in areas in which additional effort is needed, without having to move on to an advanced year inadequately prepared, or drop back and repeat an entire year.

3. The curriculum allows a considerable degree of flexibility for students with a strong commitment to research or to a particular field of medicine. In either case, participation is facilitated in relevant course work not ordinarily part of the medical curriculum, and the courses the student decides are of marginal value, even if a normal part of the curriculum, may be omitted or the information gained through other means.

4. Students may acquire material by self-directed study, if that properly meets their needs.

5. Early clinical exposure, as well as participation in special programs such as the Medical Scientist Training Program, the Neuroscience Training Program, and the Health Services Administration Program, can be accommodated easily.

6. Although it cannot be measured objectively, our curriculum undoubtedly is responsible in no small way for Stanford's success in attracting some of the most highly qualified and intellectually mature applicants. Students place an extremely high value on the opportunity to be selective, and with rare exceptions they have proven capable of assuming this responsibility. We believe this trust on the part of the faculty contributes strongly to an attitude of accountability within the student body and to the positive interaction between faculty and students.

7. Any medical curriculum must prepare college graduates to become physicians. The test of a curriculum, however, is not only that it imparts some body of knowledge, but that it instills in students a life-long commitment to the values of medicine, including the continuing acquisition and critical application of knowledge. We believe the curriculum can encourage this by placing students in a position of responsibility for their own careers from the outset.

CONCERNS ABOUT THE STANFORD
ELECTIVE CURRICULUM IN MEDICINE

1. It has been difficult to develop an effective advisory system, perhaps because of the extraordinary breadth of a medical curriculum as compared to that of a Ph.D. program. It is probable that many faculty advisors themselves have not had a sufficient understanding of the Stanford curriculum to give useful advice, and that as a result they have not been sought out by the students.

At first, medical students were assigned to advisory teams composed of several faculty members from each preclinical and clinical department and one or two upperclass medical students. When it was found that the teams and the students could never get together, advising by a pair of faculty members was substituted. Most faculty continued to be inadequately informed about the entire curriculum, however, and new students turned for advice to upperclassmen, who had personal experience, were available, and were interested, but who also had a limited understanding of the curriculum. In addition, a "sample tract" of courses was provided for preclinical students. The CCC remains divided as to whether this strengthens our curriculum by, in effect, defining a "core" of basic courses, or dilutes it.

Beginning in 1974–75, academic advising has been carried out in the Office of Student Affairs, where any student may consult one of the associate deans or any of several other faculty members who serve as academic consultants to that office. Experience in the Office of Student Affairs quickly qualifies a member of the faculty to be an effective advisor. All student study plans are submitted and monitored in that office, and those who submit questionable plans are interviewed by an associate dean. The Office of Student Affairs attempts to see every student at least once a year, as well as on any occasion a student requests advice. This approach shows promise.

2. Are we meeting our obligations to society when even a small percentage of our graduates have not had any clinical experience in, for example, psychiatry or in emergency medicine? This is a key and controversial question within the school, and it is not easily answered. We rely on the capacity of students to pass an examination in every major topic area, whether or not course work has been taken, as an indication that adequate instruction, perhaps self-instruction, has occurred. But such knowledge, even if adequate, does not take the place of experience. How useful is a clerkship experience in obstetrics or orthopedic surgery going to prove to a psychiatrist ten years after graduation? Such prefactory exposure is probably of no greater value than no experience at all. On the other hand, a great deal of time could be spent on, and resources committed to, providing each graduate with a number of such experiences. The same considerations may be argued, with the same ambiguous result, about the necessity for a rotating internship. The Stanford curriculum has the effect of moving the period at which students become responsible for their own proficiency back from the time of graduation into their years in medical school.

3. There is concern that we may be graduating a few students who have had no meaningful laboratory experience, either as undergraduates or as medical students, and who are therefore potentially deficient in their ability to critically evaluate and draw conclusions from biological experiments.

4. Given current budgetary constraints, does a medical curriculum as elective as ours make the most efficient use of faculty time and our limited clinical resources? Some data in this connection may

be of interest. Of the approximately eighty courses categorized 'as representing departmental effort, about 15 percent were not given because none was selected by students; 15 percent were selected by one to ten; 40 percent by eleven to fifty-nine; and 30 percent by sixty or more. Comparable data for courses categorized as representing individual faculty effort include: 30 percent selected by no students; 45 percent by one to ten; 25 percent by eleven to fifty-nine; and none by sixty or more. Altogether, approximately 20 percent of the courses offered attracted no students; some 25 percent of the courses were taken by fewer than ten; and only about 20 percent by sixty or more. Of the total number of clinical clerkship positions, only about 60 percent are filled. During 1974–75, one-third of our clinical clerkships were taken by only one or two students.

One can look on these data in two ways. It appears that the curriculum is associated with motivation of the faculty toward a strong teaching effort in the medical school and the university. It also seems that the elective curriculum may be inefficient, in that a good deal of faculty time goes into some courses attended by small numbers of students. Our objective, however, is to help our medical students develop attitudes and achievements that include, but are not limited to, retention of facts. Contact between faculty and individual students or small groups of students who share a common interest is more likely to promote the intellectual attainments we desire for our students than are large and efficiently organized classes.

5. Planning is difficult in a curriculum with a number of course offerings, and several constraints arise in attempting to schedule many courses at times convenient for both students and faculty. For example, when some students elect to take clinical physiology during their first year and some during their second year, then that subject must be scheduled so as not to conflict with histology (taken by almost all first-year students) or pharmacology (taken by most second-year students).

6. There are indications that increasing financial pressures felt by many medical students will in the future cause them to shorten the duration of their medical education, thus eliminating many of the options provided by the elective curriculum.

GENERAL COMMENTS

The selection of students obviously is important. The Admissions Committee puts considerable emphasis on selecting students whose records show they are independent thinkers and planners, or those who have specific goals that can be pursued better at Stanford than elsewhere. The latter often have academic plans that include involvement with other schools and departments on the university campus. The *Medical School Bulletin* states that

> A medical student wishing to derive maximum benefit from the Stanford program requires strong motivation and self-direction. The basic orientation of the school is more suitable for some students than others. We are concerned lest students arrive here and find themselves unhappy with their choice.

We admit students from a variety of academic backgrounds. For the last five admission seasons, for example, the percentage of accepted students with majors in the humanities and the social sciences has been higher than the percentage with these same backgrounds in the applicant pool.

The Fleischmann Teaching and Learning Center for self-instruction, using a variety of audiovisual aids, plays an important role in the electivity of the curriculum by providing alternatives for some courses and "supplements" to curricular offerings.

THE FUTURE OF THE ELECTIVE
MEDICAL CURRICULUM AT STANFORD

It is important to emphasize that both students and faculty are enthusiastic about the flexibility and electivity of the Stanford curriculum. When it was last extensively reviewed by the CCC and the Faculty Senate in 1973, its continuation was approved. There are, however, concerns that portend some possible modifications. The basic science subcommittee of the CCC is finding the realistic scheduling of preclinical courses increasingly difficult, and is giving consideration to defining a group of "core" preclinical courses. These will not be mandatory, but they will receive priority in scheduling. The CCC may also consider more explicit requirements for clinical clerkships, such as minimum experience in the several fields of medicine, such as surgery, psychiatry, and pediatrics. It is expected that such a relatively low degree of structure would help satisfy some of the concerns discussed in the foregoing pages, and at the same time most of the advantages of the elective curriculum.

There has been a tendency for the faculty to feel that an elective curriculum does not need close attention—indeed, that it will take care of itself through an evolutionary process based on the students' selection of courses they consider the fittest. The Darwinian approach has not, however, adequately addressed such problems as unintended duplications in and omissions from the curriculum. The Faculty Senate recently established the chairmanship of the CCC as a half-time position for a three-year renewable term. This is expected to contribute to a closer surveillance and better control of the quality of course offerings, as well as a more purposeful evaluation of the curriculum itself.

CONCLUSIONS

Although not without problems, the elective curriculum in medicine at Stanford has been very compatible with the attitudes and philosophy of the medical school and the university. We believe it has helped attract many of the most able and sophisticated students applying to study medicine. Although student attitudes, performance on national board examinations, and ratings of performance as interns are most satisfactory, they are not a measure of the success of the curriculum. Nor is it possible to estimate the cost of implementing a curriculum with this degree of flexibility. It commands a high degree of motivation on the part of faculty and students, and contributes to and relies on the resources of the entire university community. In one dimension, the curriculum differs only in extent from those at other medical schools where substantial amounts of time are left free for elective work. In another, it differs fundamentally, as there is no basic core or course that must be taken. We think perhaps its greatest strength lies in the responsibilities it places on the students. In assuming these responsibilities we hope our students acquire early the attitudes of self-direction and life-long commitment to learning. In educating the physician of tomorrow these are as important as a comprehensive exposure to currently presumed facts, many of which will too soon be obsolete.

DISCUSSION

One paradox of the elective system at Stanford is that since the majority of the students opt for courses that comprise an orthodox curriculum, why bother to have an elective system at all? While this is conceded to be an anomaly, it was still held that the elective curriculum has great value for a medical school, not least as a very effective recruiting tool.

In an elective curriculum most of the counseling is done, de facto, by upperclassmen, because with such a wide variety of courses from which to choose, the faculty is no more sophisticated about options than are the students. Thus upperclassmen are left to advise their junior counterparts on which courses are worth taking. While this has some value as a means of quality control, that is, teachers are put on the line, it does not always work to the advantage of students who need very competent counseling. More effective advisory services should be a priority in schools with elective curricula.

The discussion then turned to perceptions of efficiency in medical education. Many "bad" teachers may in fact be good with smaller groups. Unfortunately, small elective courses are viewed as inefficient, and should not be offered. The real objective should not be efficiency, but effectiveness; whatever inspires students is effective.

Cell Biology in the Curriculum*

THEODORE T. PUCK

The most common form of the American medical school curriculum includes an initial two-year period principally, but not exclusively, devoted to the basic sciences, which are taught as discrete courses in departments of anatomy, biochemistry, biophysics, biostatistics, cell biology, genetics, microbiology and immunology, pathology, pharmacology, physiology, and preventive medicine. Other basic science courses that occasionally appear in the curriculum may not be given in explicit departments.

The last two years of medical school are usually divided among the clinical departments, and administered as clerkships in each of the specialties and subspecialties of medicine. During this period the students are confronted directly with the challenge of patient care.

A variety of alternative arrangements have been proposed from time to time, such as the notable pioneering experiments carried out at Case Western Reserve, the three-year medical program, and other departures. Often, however, these new curricula fail to reflect adequately the new essential unity that has evolved in modern biological science. The resulting fragmentation deprives medical students of some of the conceptualizing power that modern developments permit; often subjects them to an unnecessary degree of detailed analysis that may rarely or never find application in their clinical training; causes repetition of some elements to a point where it is destructive of morale; and results in an unfortunate breakdown of communication between the faculties of basic science and clinical medicine. As a result, students sometimes consider the basic sciences as an empty scholastic exercise, with little relevance

* Contribution No. 221 from the Eleanor Roosevelt Institute for Cancer Research, Denver, Colorado.

to their ultimate goals in medicine, and they may become resentful and uncooperative.

It is my thesis that cell biology offers a unifying principle around which the first two years of the medical school curriculum can be built, and provides natural and powerful connections with many aspects of the clinical disciplines. Moreover, revolutions in medicine appear to be emerging that utilize the new somatic cell biology. Unless medical students are given a foundation that allows them to understand and master these developments as they emerge, we may produce physicians who are technicians, in whose hands it would be dangerous to place the great powers of the new medicine that is beginning to appear on the horizon.

Some approaches to the medical curriculum emphasize consideration of the body, organ by organ and tissue by tissue. While such analysis is vital to medical education, it should be preceded by an analysis of the cell as a functional entity. Otherwise the fundamental consideration that the body is built on the modular principle, whose fundamental unit is the cell, may be overlooked.

The body originates as a single cell, the accurate replication and genetic regulatory activity of which furnish the structure of each organ. All cells have the same total repository of information stored in their genes and chromosomes. Each differentiated cell has a particular spectrum of its genome which is active; each of the remaining genes is carefully protected from coming into a state of activity inconsistent with its particular differentiation habitus. Cells are constantly exchanging information with each other and with their fluid environment so as to maintain the dynamically poised condition required to sustain the working of the body as a whole and to continue to traverse its particular developmental cycle.

Cells are not static; they can change their differentiation state in response to information received. A normal adult liver, for example, usually has a rate of cell reproduction so low as to be almost impossible to measure. Yet extirpation of half or two-thirds of a mouse liver initiates an enormous rate of cell reproduction, which can result in restoration of the original organ in a matter of weeks. The potentiality for this action is lodged in the cells of the liver as an integral part of their structure.

A physician needs a true and deep understanding of the structure and functions of the body, as well as empathy with and sympathy for the patient as a person who requires help. The medical school must provide a conceptual framework that will be useful in both aspects of this mission. As new and revolutionary developments take place in medicine, and they certainly will in the decade ahead, this framework must be sufficiently powerful to make relatively easy the assimilation of these changes in medicine over the years.

The term genetics is sometimes used in medicine in two different ways. Its most common but limited meaning is as a synonym for heredity, and in this connection the role of genetics is conceived as the consideration of human genetic diseases—their symptomatology, treatment, and prevention, as well as affording the benefits of informed genetic counseling to affected families. The more modern implications of the term genetics include all aspects of the structure and function of the cellular genome, and the regulation of these elements so as to bring about normal or distorted patterns of differentiation and integration with the cells' surrounding structures. Thus the genetic structures and functions of somatic as well as germ cells are included.

In the proposal that follows an attempt will be made to list the concepts the medical student should have acquired by the end of his second year in medical school. It is not necessary that these be presented in a linear order. Indeed, from many points of view it would be desirable to begin the molecular approach and the approaches of gross anatomy simultaneously, in order always to keep in perspective the different levels of the body's functioning.

Many of the concepts mentioned here should have been learned by the student before coming to medical school. If he has not acquired them, however, he must be given assistance in making up such deficiencies. Finally, some consideration of the problem of sick patients should, I believe, be introduced at the very beginning of the medical curriculum, and be developed with increasing emphasis during the entire span of the medical school experience.

In his general background the entering medical student's knowledge should already encompass the necessary skills for effective communication; training in the intellectual disciplines; some understanding of human history; past and present structural principles regulating human societies; and the principal value systems professed by the world's major civilizations. He requires some understanding of the complex needs of individuals in order to maintain an active and independent life in different kinds of environments. With such a background taken for granted, a possible curriculum for the first two years could take the form to be described.

It will be obvious that most if not all of the content of the first two years of the conventional medical curriculum can be subsumed within this proposed scheme. Yet it affords the opportunity for a more tightly knit logical structure, and the ability to develop conceptual connections between parts of the medical curriculum that often are subject to artificial compartmentalization.

Different sections of this outline do not of course represent regions requiring equal amounts of time. Some of the items may be handled adequately in a paragraph or two, while others represent the content of more than one whole course. Even for schools that wish to retain the conventional curricular organization, it could be a fulfilling exercise for students to recast their informational content into a form such as the one suggested here.

OUTLINE OF PRELIMINARY PROGRAM

1. *Mathematical Review*
    a) Elements of calculus and its application to problems in medicine such as reaction velocities, kidney clearance, and growth;
    b) Elementary probability theory and its medical applications;
    c) Computer methods and their medical applications.

2. *Physical Review*
    a) Energy, potential and kinetic; the energy distribution in molecular systems;
    b) Order and disorder in molecular systems;
    c) Atomic structure and the varieties of atomic states;
    d) Molecular structure and the varieties of possible molecular states;
    e) The states of matter, and the nature of physical properties such as solubility, viscosity, and diffusion;
    f) Hydrodynamics of fluids in general, and of the circulatory system in particular. The work of the heart and the nature of hydrostatic pressure, osmotic pressure, and vapor pressure;
    g) Physical methods for study of molecular structure;
    h) Bioengineering and its applications to medicine;
    i) Interactions of radiation with nonliving and living matter;
    j) Philosophical consideration of the patient as a mechanical system on the one hand, and as a person on the other;

the need for the physician to synthesize both approaches in his dealing with patients.

3. *Chemistry, Biochemistry, and Molecular Biology*
   a) The nature of intra-atomic and intramolecular forces, and mechanisms of chemical reactions;
   b) The nature of chemical specificity;
   c) The structure of biological macromolecules and their special properties;
   d) Template or guided biosynthesis: DNA, RNA, and proteins;
   e) The synthesis structure, and dynamic actions of enzymes, antibodies, and special systems such as complement, collagen, and clotting factors;
   f) Molecular biology of cellular reactions and their interrelations;
   g) The structure, functions, and pathology of the cell membrane;
   h) A preliminary view of the actions of hormones and drugs.

4. *The Mammalian Cell as a Microorganism*
   a) The body as a modular system;
   b) The ultrastructure of cell organelles and their actions, including the cell surface, the mitochondria, the endothelial reticulum, the Golgi apparatus, the lysomes, soluble and insoluble enzymes, ribosomes and polysomes, nuclear membranes, the nucleus, and the chromosomes; the different kinds and activities of cellular RNAs; the processes of active transport, phagocytosis, pynocytosis, and excretion;
   c) The cell reproductive cycle;
   d) The variety of differentiation states of the cell;
   e) Cell genetics, genetic biochemistry, and biosynthetic pathways;
   f) Hormone receptors and hormone actions;
   g) Cell movement;
   h) The pathological states of the different cell types;
   i) Cancer and other cellular diseases;
   j) Unsolved problems of the cell in medicine.

5. *The Tissues of the Body: Cellular and Molecular Processes*
   a) Some molecular aspects of tissue differentiation and development;
   b) Cell turnover in tissues;
   c) The various roles of hormones;
   d) Cell-cell recognition phenomena;
   e) Bioelectric phenomena;
   f) Molecular aspects of tissue pathology in various diseases;
   g) The patients's subjective reactions to various kinds of tissue pathology;
   h) The role of the physician in providing accurate diagnosis, adequate information, and necessary emotional support to the patient for present problems and future developments, and therapy;
   i) Unsolved problems of tissue development and pathology

6. *Cellular and Molecular Approaches to the Organs of the Body*
   a) The body as an integrated system;
   b) The structure and function of the various communications systems utilized by the tissue and organs;
   c) The known feedback interactions and their pathologies;
   d) The action of drugs on cells, tissues, and organs, and their integration;
   e) The mind-body problem in medicine;
   f) The dynamics of healing and regeneration;
   g) Unsolved problems of organ organization and integration and its pathologies.

7. *The Whole Organism*
   a) Review of the entire human developmental process and its principal stages;
   b) The developmental and degenerative diseases, including arthritis, aging, cancer, diabetes, and the autoimmune diseases;
   c) Human emotional needs at each stage of development, and the doctor's role in assisting patients to achieve fulfillment of these needs in a fashion that maximizes the patient's total potential;
   d) The human genetic behavioral drives and their implications for medicine;
   e) Unsolved problems.

8. *The Medical Problems of Man and Society*
    A consideration of human goals and lifestyles, how they
    form and change, and their medical implications; the role of
    social pressures and institutions affecting human problems
    with which the physician must try to cope.

Physiology in the Curriculum

D. HAROLD COPP

INTRODUCTION

Although Aristotle and Galen were both interested in biological function, the term "physiology" was first introduced in 1554 by the distinguished French physician Jean Fernel in his treatise *De Naturale Parte Medicinae*. In it he divided medicine into three major topics: *physiologia* (dealing with function), *pathologia* (dealing with disease), and *therapeutica* (dealing with clinical medicine). These are still major subjects in the medical school curriculum, even though the boundaries may be blurred in the integrated systems approach to training. Much of the physiology described by Fernel was based largely on gross anatomy, and bore little resemblance to modern physiology. Indeed a knowledge of structure and ultrastructure is essential to the understanding of biological functions. The foundations for modern physiology were laid by William Harvey some seventy years later, with the publication of his treatise, *Exercitatio anatomica de motu cordis et sanguinis in animalibus,* in which he described the first application of experimental method to the study of function. In his introduction there is a statement that would strike a familiar note to a student in first-year physiology today:

> When I first tried animal experimentation for the purpose of discovering the motions and functions of the heart by actual inspection and not by other people's books, I found it so truly difficult that I almost believed with Fracastorius, that the motion of the heart was to be understood by God alone.

Harvey's work opened up the scientific approach to problems in human biology and led to the great conceptual advances of the nineteenth and twentieth centuries. Among these can be included

151

Claude Bernard's emphasis on the importance of the constancy
of the environment; Walter Cannon's concept of homeostasis; and
the principle of dynamic equilibrium introduced by Rudolf Schoen-
heimer.

PHYSIOLOGY IN THE CURRICULUM

Naturally I subscribe to Fernel's view of the importance of physiology in medical training, whether taught as a separate subject or
as part of an integrated program. Edra L. and Helen W. Spilman
made a recent study of the attitudes of medical students and staff at
Mount Sinai School of Medicine in New York City on the relevance
of nine basic science courses.[1] Most medical students, interns, residents, and clinical faculty rated physiology most relevant, with
pathology close behind. Strangely enough, first-year students rated
physiology somewhere in the middle, just above gross anatomy; in
succeeding years, however, physiology rose to a much higher level
than the other basic medical sciences. Realization of the relevance
of the subject evidently increases as the students are exposed to
clinical problems.

For this reason it is important that instruction in physiology be
introduced early in the medical student's career, preferably in the
first year of training. It has even been suggested that physiology
should be moved back a year and made a premedical requirement,
as has occurred in some schools in the case of biochemistry. I
consider this a backward step. Large science courses in physiology
are no substitute for the intensive and clinically oriented presentation in medical school.

A second approach is the use of a common "core" basic science
course for all students of the health sciences. When this was tried
at Laval University it proved disastrous. Aside from the drawback
of the large classes involved, the varied preparations, motivations,
and backgrounds of the students make it difficult to give a course
that rises above the lowest common denominator. It is my personal
view that instruction in the various health professions schools should
be tailored to those specific students.

I should mention, however, that at the University of British
Columbia we give the same basic science courses to first-year
dentistry and medical students. Although the dental students sometimes complain about being taught unnecessary anatomy and physiology, the common learning experience has raised the standards

in the School of Dentistry, and the graduates in both medicine and dentistry have a much greater respect for and understanding of each other's profession.

A second important consideration is the continued input of physiology in the clinical years of training. This can be accomplished by participation in ward rounds and operating theater clinics, and by the introduction of elective courses in applied physiology in the upper years.

THE UNIVERSITY OF BRITISH COLUMBIA PROGRAM

In organizing instruction in physiology it is essential that both faculty and students have a clear idea of the objectives of the course—both general and specific. In common with a number of other schools we have prepared a statement of educational objectives, based on that developed by the physiology department at the University of Aarhus in Denmark (it is modified for laboratory work). The introductory statement is as follows:

> With clearly stated and detailed objectives, it will be possible for us to experiment with self-instruction in the future. The fall term will consist of an initial introductory survey course consisting of 30 lectures and 15 practical exercises. This will be optional for those who already have previous training in physiology or who wish to follow a program of health instruction. There will be non-credit evaluation tests at the beginning and at the end of the course and the second major part of the course will be systems oriented with a heavy emphasis on practical applications in medicine, and to a limited extent in dentistry.

There has been a tendency in many places to reduce or eliminate the time spent in laboratory work in physiology. At British Columbia we belong to the old school. We feel that one learns by doing, and that it is better for students to gain experience in the handling of living tissues and animals in the laboratory, rather than to obtain their first, and possibly disastrous, experience with patients. It is essential, however, that the laboratory experiments meet certain criteria: they must illustrate important principles or techniques; they must be relevant to future career needs; and above all they must work.

Another benefit accrues from practical experience, whether in the laboratory or in demonstrations, and that is the opportunity for contacts and discussions between faculty and students in small groups. We also rate as practical work the tutorials and seminars in which the students take an active part in the preparation and presentation of materials. While it is not our intention to turn the students into physiologists or scientists, we do feel they should know the limitations of experimental methods that give rise to new knowledge, and be able to assess the validity of reports appearing in the literature. In this regard we conduct tutorials in which the students discuss published reports of research findings and critically evaluate the results thereof. It is perhaps significant of student attitudes at British Columbia that over 80 percent of the entering students in 1975 chose to take laboratory in the first term, even though it was an elective.

STAFFING PROBLEMS

Traditionally, departments of physiology have been staffed primarily by medically qualified teachers in this subject, so fundamental to the practice of medicine. Unfortunately, the present economic differential has made it increasingly difficult to recruit M.D.'s for graduate work or research or for subsequent academic careers in physiology. This is to be regretted, because such teachers are able to provide a better integration between the science and application of physiology. We hope this situation may be corrected, in part by cross-appointments between the Department of Physiology and clinical departments, and by the involvement of clinical teachers in certain aspects of the physiology course.

CONCLUSION

My attitude toward the role of physiology is somewhat conservative because British Columbia is a traditional medical school where departments still retain the primary responsibility for teaching. For many years we have had a very successful integrated course in the neurological sciences, involving neuroanatomy, neurophysiology, and clinical neurology. We are also planning an integrated course in endocrinology, which will cover anatomy, biochemistry, and physiology and medicine. The success of any training program, however, depends upon the effectiveness and enthusiasm of the faculty, and the motivation and capabilities of the students. In both respects we feel we are fortunate.

Note

1. Edra L. Spilman and Helen W. Spilman, "A Pair Comparison Study of the Relevance of Nine Basic Science Courses," *Journal of Medical Education,* 50, no. 7 (1975): 667–72.

DISCUSSION

In reply to a question, Copp stated that a small committee of faculty members and students developed the educational objectives for the University of British Columbia program. Instruction can be tailored to the needs of the individual. During the first term, for example, both classroom and laboratory time are optional, although laboratory is mandatory in the second term. The only requirement is that students meet the educational objectives of the program.

A difficult problem for any medical school dean is how to attract the best physiologists to his faculty, and how to keep them interested in teaching medical students. Copp noted that, at British Columbia, teacher performance is given a great deal of weight when promotions are being considered, and there is a monthly student evaluation of the quality of instruction. If a faculty member receives a low rating, he may not teach.

Pathology in the Curriculum

DONALD W. KING

PATHOLOGY IN THE UNITED STATES

Pathology has long been considered the introduction-to-medicine course and a major foundation of the medical school curriculum. Formerly a pathology course consisted of some two hundred to four hundred contact hours of instruction; more recently several major alterations in time and structure have been introduced. Pathology is now often compressed into seventy-five to one hundred and fifty hours in the first year, and/or combined into pathophysiology courses with clinical departments in the second and third years.

Traditionally, the first part of the pathology course (general pathology or principles of pathology) consisted of lectures in cell injury, inflammation, immunology, genetic diseases, neoplasia, infectious disease, and aging. This sequence has, however, been fragmented, splintered, and diminished by the development of new courses and new departments. Many schools now have separate courses in genetics and immunology; infectious disease has been split between pathology, microbiology, medicine, and pediatrics; and cell injury is partly covered in cell biology courses. More recently, stimulated by the formation of cancer centers, distinct courses in neoplasia have begun to appear in the clinical years. Systemic pathology, a careful review of organ and system pathology, has either been compressed in the first year or integrated as pathophysiology courses in the third or fourth clinical years, with varying degrees of success.

Nevertheless, pathology textbooks, as with textbooks of medicine, pediatrics, and biochemistry, represent the basic fundamental core of science knowledge presented in an organized fashion in the majority of medical schools in this country. The integration of

156

courses, rather than the production of integrated textbooks, has instead usually resulted in multiple, voluminous syllabi, often verbose, poorly written, and poorly illustrated, and containing individual classifications and organizational patterns accepted only on a local basis.

Regardless of the number of hours and the variations in curricula, pathology courses have remained as standard as any course in the medical school. Since they represent an introduction to medicine, they have of necessity continued to cover the complete disease spectrum in an organized manner.

PATHOLOGY AT COLUMBIA UNIVERSITY

The pathology course at Columbia University medical school consists of 163 contact-hours, with approximately sixty hours of laboratory, and forty of discussion time. Utilizing some one hundred and forty instructors for a combined medical-dental graduate student body of about two hundred and fifteen, it has been possible to split up the class into discussion and laboratory groups of fifteen to eighteen students, and elective seminar groups of six to eight.

In a two-week Introductory Survey Course, the complete spectrum of pathology is presented in a syllabus containing some two hundred and forty instructional objectives and about three hundred individual microphotographs on microfiche (Figure 1).

Each year an experimental group of ten medical students has elected to take part in a special program, utilizing their laboratory and seminar time (one hundred hours with one instructor) while continuing to attend all lectures and to take examinations. For the past three years, each year a different program has been set up for this group, concentrating on developing slide-tape presentations, student-author computer programs, and videotape presentations.

In the first year, the students prepared six slide-tape presentations, two in each subject, including programs in immunology, chemical carcinogenesis, and virology. A fifteen- or twenty-minute slide-tape presentation on these subjects involved library research and the preparation of slides and a script. The total cost for each program was approximately $25.00. After review, the programs were made available in the library for the entire class (Figure 2).

In this connection, incidentally, at the Given Institute of Pathobiology in Aspen, a small group of faculty members from various schools initiated the production of similar slide-tape programs for

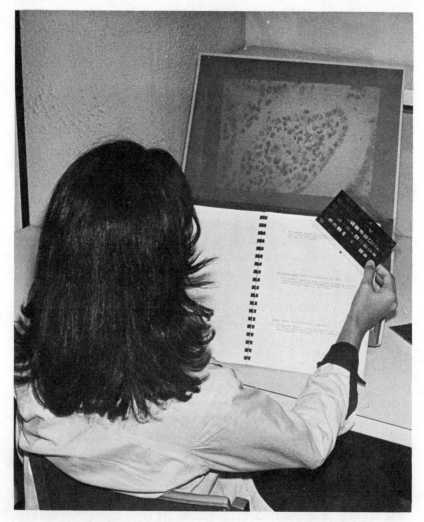

Figure 1. A Student Participates in the Introductory Survey Course in Pathology at Columbia University.

national distribution. Rolla Hill of the Department of Pathology, State University of New York at Syracuse, with a group of pathologists and the cooperation of the National Audiovisual Center, completed several such programs on immunology, kidney, and gastrointestinal and pulmonary pathology, which are now avail-

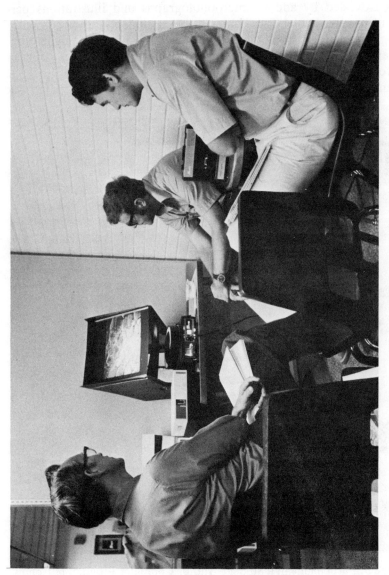

Figure 2. A Slide-Tape Presentation in the Library of Columbia University.

able for use throughout the country at $17.50 each. The cost for developing each program was approximately $1,500.

In the second year at Columbia, a computer program—the CASE system developed at the University of Illinois by William Harless— was extended by adding microphotographs and illustrations pertinent to a particular case. Later, using a student-author computer program on loan from the Hewlitt Packer Company, eight computer microphotograph packages were developed in the area of systemic pathology (Figure 3).

In the 1974–75 academic year, twelve students prepared six

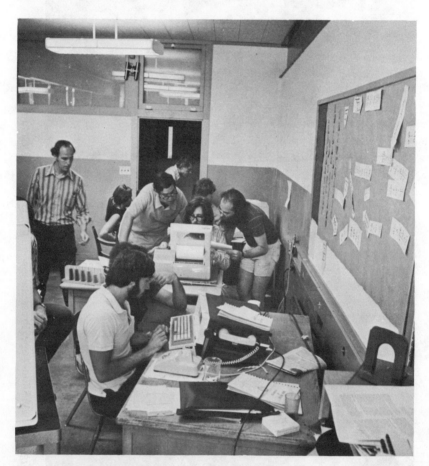

Figure 3. Participants in a Student-Author Computer Program at Columbia University.

videotape presentations of clinical pathological conferences on a specific subject. Faculty members prepared six-minute video introductions to each laboratory session, allowing for a uniformity of the material being presented in ten different laboratory sections.

Finally, an undergraduate program in pathology has been developed at Columbia College, similar to that developed at the University of Colorado several years ago, in which general pathology is taught to graduate students in the main university, as well as to junior and senior undergraduates. A full four-credit-hour course with sixty contact hours in pathobiology is given every other year; it covers immunology, genetics, cell injury, inflammation, and neoplasia. Comparative examinations have shown that students in the junior and senior years of college are able to encompass the same amount of material as a freshman or sophomore in the medical school. The one defect is that many of them have not had courses in histology and do less well in the identification of microscopic lesions.

This year a complete pathology course of 180 hours is being proposed for third-year undergraduate students in the biomedical program at the City University of New York. After completing the fourth year as undergraduates, including the equivalent of the first two years of medical school, the students will be admitted to the third year of one of six or seven medical schools in the New York area. Much of the material presented to this class will be taught by the use of closed circuit, whereby live and cassette videotapes of gross conference, microscopic and research seminars will be transmitted by microwave (Figure 4).

SUGGESTIONS FOR THE FUTURE

The teaching of pathology in the medical curriculum, along with other courses, is undergoing an appreciable change as a result of an overcrowded curriculum; the introduction of new courses; the emphasis on health care delivery; the change from a four- to a three-year curriculum; the increase in the number of electives; the reevaluation and often complete elimination of laboratory time; the substitution of the pass-fail grading system; the development of independent study groups; the question of relevance in the curriculum; the introduction of students on curriculum committees; and the deemphasis of basic science.

Pathology has come to play a much larger role in the chemical

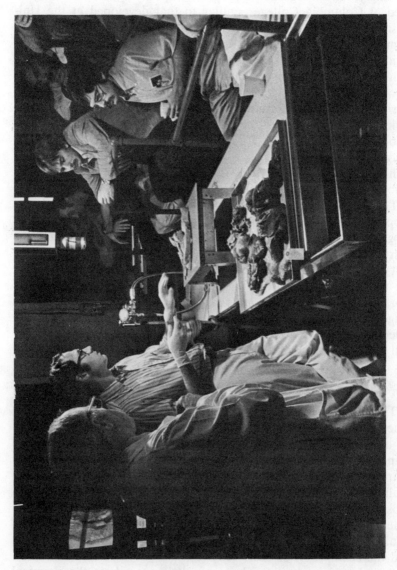

Figure 4. Material Presented to a Class Being Transmitted by Closed-Circuit Microwave.

laboratory, in program and center grants, and in integration of the teaching of clinical subspecialties. While its role in the clinical area has been markedly expanding, its role in basic science has diminished, due to lack of funds, space, curriculum time, and research interest on the part of students and residents. Professors of pathology must adjust to their changing roles and to the different objectives of the medical schools. In addition to accepting its new clinical responsibilities, pathology should become heavily involved in M.D.–Ph.D. programs.

The United States has embarked on the training of large numbers of new physicians, emphasizing the provision of health care services, even though a practical, innovative system has not yet been worked out. The concepts of science, as the basis of medicine and science for science itself, are disappearing. While it is impossible in this short space to document fully the relevance of science to the practice of medicine, it is not an act of faith, and this is, I think, generally accepted by most medical faculties. It will be many years before the realization sets in that the physicians of the future may be less able to cope with new advances in the biosciences as a result of their lack of background in the basic sciences. This depressing fact may be mitigated by the development of peer review processes, which may force physicians to review the basic sciences more extensively once they have graduated from medical school, but the depth or value of continuing education programs has yet to be determined.

I would urge that medical school pathology departments, in order to protect their future faculty members, promote, encourage, and expand to the greatest degree possible the development of M.D.–Ph.D. programs, so that at least 5 percent of the student body continues to undergo the rigorous disciplinary education that was once demanded of every medical student. This is not to denigrate or minimize the importance of health care delivery systems, or the necessity to provide better health care for every American citizen. Rather, in order to protect the health program twenty-five years in the future, we should insist that a small percentage of our graduates continue to receive a heavy science background so they may readily incorporate new scientific knowledge into the practice of medicine. Medical economics, medical administration, behavioral sciences, and emergency room medicine are all subjects that can be best taught during the residency; they should not further restrict or act as substitutes for the basic science components of the medical school curriculum.

One may never return to the past. The country and the medical schools are committed to the development of primary care practitioners and to the redistribution and despecialization of physicians. Nevertheless, we in pathology and other departments in the medical school should accept a new committment: to encourage at least 5 percent of our student body to participate in expanded basic science M.D.–Ph.D. programs, so that upcoming faculty and leaders in health will be well prepared for the future.

DISCUSSION

The audiovisual method of instruction described by King was felt to be a valuable development, and it should be adopted more widely. At present only six other medical schools have similar projects underway.

New Directions in Medical Education: Primary Care*

JOEL J. ALPERT

Most medical training, both undergraduate and postgraduate, is now provided in large academic medical centers which specialize in providing complex, subspecialty care. As a result of the presentation of this type of practice as an occupational model, many medical students come to believe that tertiary care and modern medicine are synonomous and that modern medicine can only be practiced in association with a large urban hospital. The current medical model also leads to the overproduction of specialists at the expense of primary care physician output. Several studies indicate that the primary care physician is more likely to locate in an area remote from an academic medical center. Although available data do not show direct correlation, the current emphasis on subspecialty training with its dependence on tertiary care centers mitigates against the dispersal of such physicians into medically underserved areas.[1]

This statement, taken from the report of the House Interstate and Foreign Commerce Committee on the Health Manpower Bill, carries a simple and direct message. Primary medical care is of great concern to the Congress. While this concern extends to specialty distribution, it is largely expressed in terms of the geographic maldistribution of physicians.

Beginning with legislative developments serves to emphasize that planning for primary care education is no longer the sole responsibility of medical schools. Congress, at least in the House version of the manpower bill, has selected family practice as the basic primary care discipline, and in this respect may be initiating the development of a defined primary care service. Legislative bodies

*This work has been supported in part by the Robert Wood Johnson Foundation and by contract #NO1–PE–34074 of the Department of Health, Education, and Welfare.

can address the primary care problem by specifying the location of practice opportunities, by limiting entry into hospital-based specialty positions, and by selective funding of programs.

Educators should not accept the selection of a single primary care model uncritically. While we must recognize the force of society exercising its desires through the legislative process, we should approach a single solution cautiously, since single solutions are not consistent with the needs of this country.

The appropriate primary care practice model will very likely vary from one community to another. Rural areas may require one model and urban centers something very different. While outside funds specifically earmarked for primary care education serve as a stimulus for the medical school to define where its primary care commitments lie, one hopes the choice will continue with the individual medical school.

Educators must address the educational mismatch that has, unfortunately, characterized medical education since the Flexner report.[2] This mismatch includes the failure to consider that most graduates practice some form of primary care, and to the failure to address the fact that medical education has been dominated by the teaching hospital staffed by specialists.[3] While this situation has yielded many benefits, its exclusiveness may be substantially credited for the development of the present severe shortage of primary care practitioners.

With this introduction, let me now move on to trends in undergraduate education for primary care. I will first present a definition of primary care, then briefly review the history of undergraduate programs in primary care, and, finally, offer a suggested plan for primary care education in the fifteen years ahead.

WHAT IS PRIMARY CARE?

Primary care can be defined as being within the personal rather than the public health system, and is therefore focused on the health needs of individuals and families [4]—it is family-oriented. Primary care is "first contact" care, and thus should be separated from secondary care and tertiary care, which are based on referral rather than initial contact.

Primary care assumes longitudinal responsibility for the patient regardless of the presence or absence of disease. The primary care physician holds the contract for providing personal health services over a period of time. Specifically, primary care is neither limited to the course of a single episode of illness nor confined to the ambulatory setting. It serves as the "integrationist" for the patient. When other health resources are involved, the primary care physician retains the coordinating role. He or she cares for as many of the patient's problems as possible, and, where referral is indicated, fulfills his longitudinal responsibility as the integrationist.

Some would suggest that primary care ought to end when the patient is hospitalized, and that ambulatory care could then be said to equal primary care. Many medical problems that require secondary services are largely treated on an ambulatory basis, however, with only occasional hospitalization. Conversely, the decision to hospitalize a patient may sometimes be based on psychosocial factors in management rather than on medical complexity. There is, in addition, strong support for the view that the physician who practices ambulatory and hospital medicine is a better physician than the one who practices only ambulatory medicine. For these reasons, the site of care alone, whether hospital, home, or office, is an insufficient base for a definition of primary care.

By this definition, most internists, pediatricians, and family physicians are primary care practitioners. By this definition, most of the physicians in these three clinical disciplines can be expected to continue to practice primary care. They will undoubtedly do this in teams with other health professionals, and in groups rather than as solo practitioners.

A BRIEF HISTORICAL OVERVIEW

The closest medical education has come to any program for general practice was in the first part of this century, when undergraduate education followed by a rotating internship constituted sufficient preparation. The proliferation of medical specialties totally changed this situation. Many programs that may be identified as primary care efforts were not directed at preparation for practice. These were attempts to improve the hospital care of patients,[5] such as introducing follow-up to hospital care,[6] or to reverse the fragmentation of care in the outpatient department.[7] These programs focused largely on the psychological and social aspects of medicine, exposing students to only limited aspects of primary care. As far as past programs are concerned, there was no broadly conceived framework to provide a base for describing undergraduate primary care, nor any demonstration of a unique body of knowledge.

Only a limited number of places existed where primary care, as defined, could be taught. The physician's office, the patient's home, and the hospital were the principal locations. The goals of most of the programs appear to have been determined largely by the physical site of the program, rather than by any major philosophical view. Programs in outpatient departments in various hospitals, for example, had much more in common than did programs within one institution, but located in different areas.

Generally, programs in primary care sought to foster what may be called positive attitudes toward patients, families, and colleagues. Areas of program concern included the physician-patient relationship, teamwork, the appropriate use of consultants, and recordkeeping. Internal medicine, pediatrics, surgery, obstetrics, and psychiatry were the clinical clerkships in which these skills and attitudes could be taught. Psychosomatic problems and chronic illnesses were seen as the clinical problems where these skills were most needed and could be applied.

The first identified site of primary care education was the physician's office, where the practitioner was the student's preceptor. Preceptorships have never been a major consideration in the United States, at least in terms of curriculum time, and yet in other areas of the world they appear to play a useful role in medical education. Perhaps the lack of interest in this country can be explained by the absence of a defined general practitioner service, since the preceptorship for the most part has been associated with general practice. Preceptorships have largely been ignored by the academic medical centers, despite reports of success as measured by student and preceptor enthusiasm. The most popular experiences appear to have been in rural practices.[8]

Another place is the patient's home. Home care programs were largely developed in the United States, most often originating in the hospital out of a concern to initiate follow-up for previously hospitalized patients.[9] Originally home care programs, in general, dealt with episodes of illness rather than with continuity of care. The faculty, being hospital-based, was too often still in training and inexperienced with respect to care outside the hospital. In almost all of the programs the patients were indigent and often elderly.

Home care programs may have demonstrated to students the value of going into the patient's home, but there is no evidence that they benefited from the experience. The home is obviously important as a site of health care, both for episodes of illness and for continuing care. Like the preceptorship, home care belongs in any fully developed program of primary care, but as a part of an overall program, not as a single or isolated activity.

Ambulatory services in the hospital are said to most closely approach a primary care setting.[10] These services were originally planned as consultative or secondary care clinics, however, in addition to providing emergency care.

Almost all ambulatory programs that attempted to improve primary care teaching were faced initially with the need to reorganize the hospital outpatient departments, which suffered because of their inability to alter in any major way their relationships with inpatient services. But changing the organization of an outpatient clinic did not transform it into a place to deal with common disorders as long as the relationship between physician and patient was disease-oriented. The faculty were primarily specialists and subspecialists, and the influence of specialty organizations and of finding disease was overwhelming. Even those students who expressed an interest in working in the outpatient department dealt almost exclusively with a disadvantaged population, as they did in home care programs.

Comprehensive and family care programs were also developed in the outpatient setting, because as experiments in medical education they were part of the curriculum.[11] Most faculty members were unwilling to recognize these programs as representing any major commitment on the part of the medical schools, however, and participating students often found themselves in a position of conflict between family care activities and the scheduled medical course. When students volunteered, this conflict was not a significant factor, but when they were assigned for experimental purposes, major antagonisms and resistance arose.

The experiences of some students left them impressed with the negative aspects of primary care, and this view was reinforced by the majority of the faculty. Certainly the programs did not influence students to select primary care careers. But they did teach continuity, did focus on first contact outside of the hospital, and the student was placed in the position of providing health as well as illness care for a family.

The family care and comprehensive care programs emphasized the importance of the family as the unit of health care, and of the contribution that can be made by the primary care physician. Fundamental for future planning were such observations as: 1) the introduction of these programs in the fourth year came too late to affect student goals; [12] 2) the student needed an experience of at least six months; [13] 3) student knowledge compared with that acquired in a traditional clerkship was similar; and 4) there were some risks involved in introducing such experiences too early in medical school.[14]

MODELS FOR PRIMARY CARE

A number of new places where educational models for primary care can be developed are now being emphasized. One of the requirements of the American Board of Family Practice, for example, is that there be a model practice if there is to be an accredited residency program. The model practice is also being developed in programs in internal medicine and pediatrics, but most of these are not available to medical students. In retrospect, the more successful family care programs appear to have functioned as model practices.[15]

A recurrent theme in all of these efforts has been the conflict between the goals of any primary care program and the goals of hospital medicine. This theme expresses itself in a number of ways. When the preclinical student, who has participated with some enthusiasm in a primary care program, arrives on the ward and comes face-to-face with hospital medicine, he may find himself in disagreement with his intern when his primary care responsibility conflicts with his ward duties. It is also seen when a faculty member joins a resident in belittling the referring physician. Not only do faculty members fail to present the student with satisfactory primary care models, but very few residents offer models of the primary care resident in training. Thus the student identifies with his intern and resident, and his primary care interest is overwhelmed by the demands of hospital medicine. If this situation is to be avoided, the student needs a model of a practicing primary care physician, as well as of a resident preparing for such a career.

A series of reports in the mid-1960s called for a national commitment to the education of personal, primary, or family physicians. Perhaps the most important, the Millis Report, called for extension of university control to include graduate (residency) training, and for a national obligation to produce primary care physicians.[16]

Also in the 1960s, poverty was "rediscovered," and the spiraling costs of medical care forced the nation to reexamine its medical priorities. Among the results were a slowdown of the research effort and the involvement of the federal government in many large-scale service programs. Academic faculty came to the realization that continued funding for research was not a natural law.

Medical schools and teaching hospitals, confronted with a population that used their facilities for primary care, but at the same time received generally inadequate health care, became engaged in neighborhood health centers, young people's programs, and maternal and infant health projects.

New medical schools were established in response to the acknowledged manpower crisis caused by the inadequate number and unequal distribution of physicians. General practitioners were not being replaced by younger physicians, and in the ghettos of large cities there were almost no primary practitioners to meet the needs of the disadvantaged population; the rural areas had none.

The admission by educators of the need for primary care training courses was undoubtedly a necessary first step. There was no evidence, however, that the new schools would actually produce primary care practitioners. Clearly the charge was unlikely to succeed without a major change in the climate of the medical schools.

What is the current situation in academic medical centers? S. A. Schroeder in 1974 reported on a survey of 93 percent of the academic medical centers in this country.[17] It supported the general impression that there has been intense activity in the development of primary care programs: half the centers had made major changes in the preceding two years. It was noted that minimal curriculum time had been devoted to teaching ambulatory care to undergraduate students, and that the ambulatory care population was heavily weighted with the urban poor. Two-thirds of the centers were training new health practitioners; half had developed courses for graduate training in family practice; and another quarter were planning such programs. There was little mention of how the other clinical departments were involved in primary care programs, how they were reordering priorities, or how they were allocating resources.

Governance for the development of the programs described, was widely dispersed in a variety of forms. In short Schroeder's report suggested that the history of primary care was repeating itself, in that most medical schools as of 1974 had not made a major effort to promote primary care education.

A PLAN FOR PRIMARY CARE EDUCATION

Part of the failure to accord a high enough priority to primary care education is that it has not been a main commitment of the medical schools. Just as medical education and medical research compete for finite resources at the public level, so primary care must compete for finite educational resources at the medical school level. When the time comes to select medical students and to allocate curriculum time, no one speaks up loudly and consistently for the needs of the student who will enter primary care. There are exceptions of course. In many schools family practice has assumed this role. Often the other clinical departments, particularly internal medicine and pediatrics, are sufficiently interested in this issue to be unwilling to relinquish responsibility to the new department of family medicine, but not concerned enough to develop effective educational programs. The result can be conflict, lack of a program, or a diluted effort to implement one.

What are the obligations of the clinical departments to primary care? All medical school departments ought to have a stake in any program that should account for the majority of graduates. Those specialities that have important but presently ill-defined roles in primary care—such as psychiatry, obstetrics and gynecology, and community medicine—must join pediatrics, internal medicine, and family practice in developing the school's program. The optimal solution may be an interdisciplinary effort with the participation of all departments, but not dependent on any single one.

Primary care needs to establish ties with other health science fields, particularly nursing and social service. At present the relative roles of the physician, nurse, and social worker in primary care are in flux. Communication among these disciplines is essential as new programs emerge.

What specific elements within educational programs are required for primary care? The five ingredients are, specifically, the *students,* the *faculty,* the *patients,* the *curriculum* structure, and the *setting.*

They are all related, each affecting the other to form the "learning environment."

Students are the most important ingredient in medical education. Is it possible that students now accepted in medical school are those least likely to pursue primary care careers? And, if so, can this be changed? In general, those accepted are more likely to have majored in the sciences, to have had high scores on their Medical College Admission Tests, and to have had high grades in college. They have usually attended private rather than public universities, and overrepresent the middle- and upper-middle-classes.

Yet the majority of these students, at least on entering medical school, have indicated a desire to pursue primary care careers. As seniors, however, their career choices have been definitely directed toward the specialties. Their interest in a career in primary care has not been sufficiently strong to counter the pressures to specialize that exist within the medical education experience. Specialties were presented as career options, but no identified careers were presented as opportunities in primary care.

Might students less scientifically oriented have pursued primary care careers? And what about those underrepresented in medical school, such as blacks, women, and the poor? Might these students have resisted the pressures to specialize?

It has been suggested that one way to get primary physicians is to recruit just these groups. For example, black and economically disadvantaged students may return to their communities as primary care practitioners; the disadvantaged could not afford to specialize; women might be attracted to pediatrics and family medicine. Such a student body would be more humanistic, more representative, and less scientific. There is no evidence, however, that these students possess those characteristics, or, if they do, would become primary care physicians if exposed to the same medical experience as their colleagues and predecessors. Moreover, although no major changes were made in the selection process, students in the 1960s began to express a definite interest in primary care.[18] There was a talented and committed group of students that showed every sign of seeking careers in primary care.

A good primary care program requires a good *faculty*. In a number of programs the faculty are not, have been never, or have ceased to be, engaged in primary practice. It would certainly be incongruous for cardiologists to teach their skills to students and house staff without having practiced cardiology. Students are quick to perceive this inconsistency. The implication seems to be that primary medical practice is a less demanding field that can be taught adequately by specialists or nonpractitioners. This also assumes that primary care practice is equal to the sum of several specialists' practices. Primary care programs need primary care faculty, and the shortage of such talented and qualified faculty must be addressed. Training programs should be developed both for those in practice and those completing residencies.

One problem in faculty selection is the issue of academic rank and promotion. Should primary care teachers be judged on the same basis as their research colleagues, namely, on the quantity and quality of their research, on their participation in learned societies, and their teaching responsibilities and skills? This is part of the larger issue of the relative merits of teaching versus research that concerns most university faculties; it should not present any special or unique problems for the primary care faculty. They can do research, and have a responsibility to do so, but the volume of research publications must be balanced against other factors when it comes time for promotion.

Patients are more of an influential factor in primary care than in secondary or tertiary care. They are having an increasing voice in whether or not they wish to participate in teaching, and greater recognition is being given to patients' rights.

It is obvious that patient contact is essential in any primary care program. Although concern has been expressed about the acceptability of students to patients in the primary care setting, it has been our experience that, with tact and honesty, patients of all economic classes accept the physician-in-training if they are assured that he is adequately supervised, and if their right to change physicians is respected.

Primary care educational programs should ideally introduce the student in a variety of roles to a variety of patients. The programs should direct or be affiliated with primary care units that have organizational and patient diversity at different levels of development. That is the laboratory, the case material of primary care, just as patients with various kinds of arthritis make up the caseload of a rheumatology trainee. If primary care education is indeed the central philosophy of the program, this orientation is a natural one—a core training in primary care with specialty experience selectivity added, not the reverse.

An adequate amount of *curriculum time* must be devoted to primary care education, but, perhaps more important, the time must be arranged appropriately within the curriculum in all four years of medical school. The present situation of considerable elective time provides that opportunity.

While the goal is not to give the student experience with every problem he will face in practice, there is a need to convey to him the sense of how a range of problems arise, evolve, and resolve, so that he does not assume a short-term view. Moreover, all these content areas cannot be experienced in one year. Some require more clinical maturity and "readiness" on the part of the student if they are to have their maximum impact.

In general, programs in medical education have emphasized block, short-term experiences at the expense of longitudinal ones; this has been detrimental to specialty as well as to primary care education. The management of several chronic disease patients through acute crises, for example, is not the educational equivalent of managing one such patient over a period of time. Both experiences have educational value.

Developing a curriculum with this concept in mind poses a number of practical problems. How is continuity meshed with rotation through other services or in other hospitals? Equally difficult for students, particularly at earlier stages of development, is the problem of coping with the change of pace required in moving from acute care, where the basic need is to extract information quickly, to the management of long-term illnesses, where a different interview manner and relationship with the patient is required.

During medical school the student has not been shown that different situations may require different or more flexible techniques of patient work-up. The student must learn that although a complete work-up rarely fits the clinical situation, there is insufficient guidance to help him devise a suitable model for the more common, brief, but long-term contact he will have with patients.

Undergraduates should begin medical school with exposure to and contact with patients whose needs are in the primary care area. The curriculum must emphasize primary care, must provide allotted time in all four years, and must be supported by the overall medical school experience.

Such a program, beginning in the first year, would include formal course work, an introduction to interviewing techniques, and a weekly preceptor experience. Formal course work could cover human development and health services research delivery, and a coordinated offering of courses usually taught by departments of psychiatry, community medicine, and preventive medicine.

Year two might include field experiences in home care programs and assignment either as a participant or observer, the latter towards the end of the year. Exposure should occur in primary care settings, such as neighborhood health centers and physicians' offices, and there could be additional formal course work. Year two, but more likely year three, would see most students accepting longitudinal clinical responsibility in a primary care program, which may also function as the university's primary care laboratory. Year four, which in most schools is elective, might provide the student with preceptorship experience for one month or longer. Schools could develop an integrated six-month clinical clerkship in primary care, while continuing the longitudinal experience into the fourth year. Clinical rotations should also be available in neighborhood health centers or community hospitals, but no clerkship should be offered in places that lack a committed and identified faculty.

The final ingredient is the *setting* of the primary care education program, specifically, its size, organization, and relationship to secondary and tertiary care systems and to the patient population; the setting is crucial to the success of the primary care curriculum. For example, the work setting, which for medical education has been the hospital, has obviously had a major influence on educational programs.

Schools of medicine should thus become involved in many settings geared to primary care, especially outside the hospital—neighborhood health centers, physicians' offices, health maintenance organizations, and group practices—where they should conduct education and research.

SUMMARY

A rapid increase in the number of primary care practitioners is what society indicates it wants, and influences outside the medical education system may be all that is required to effect such a change. A shift in terms of financial support to education, directed specifically to this end, changes in the medical practice system, and some limitation on the availability of subspecialty careers would probably have the desired effect. Not only should more practitioners be prepared, however, but they should be better educated for practice. To accomplish this aim, certain changes in medical education are recommended, including:

1. An acknowledgement by the university of its role in coordinating primary care education at the medical school, graduate, and continuing education levels. For example, while modifying undergraduate education, there must be visible residency programs in primary care.

2. The medical school must set as a priority the development of criteria for selecting students who will be suitable candidates for careers in primary medicine practice.

3. A primary care education program should be developed within each medical school.

4. The obligations of specialty clinical departments to primary care education must be defined. These departments in the past have correctly considered the development of their own disciplines as a priority. At present, however, there is an important gap between the body of knowledge and techniques of specialty medicine and how they can and should be applied at the primary care level. The fact that, short of a major revolution in the way medicine is practiced, most physicians in training will end up in primary care practice underscores the importance of utilizing appropriate aspects of all of medicine in primary care practice.

5. The university should develop sites for primary care education. In selecting programs to establish or to become affiliated with, a diversity of patient population and practice organizations should be sought. Together, these settings should be considered a part of the university's medical effort.

In short, the medical education organization, which includes the medical school, its parent university, and the teaching hospital, has important work to do. At present there is a good deal of uncertainty as to how we ought to provide quality primary medical care to this nation. This very uncertainty provides a climate in which change is possible, and in which education for primary care in the medical school can be improved dramatically.

Notes

1. U.S. Congress, House, Committee on Interstate and Foreign Commerce, *Health Manpower of 1975, Report No. 94–266,* 94th Cong., 1st sess., 7 June (Washington: U.S. Government Printing Office): 26.
2. J. Jason, "The Relevance of Medical Education to Medical Practice," *Journal of the American Medical Association* 212, no. 12 (1970): 2092–95.

3. R. Stevens, *American Medicine and the Public Interest* (New Haven: Yale University Press, 1971).

4. J. J. Alpert and E. Charney, *The Education of Physicians for Primary Care*, DHEW Publ. No. (HRA) 75–3113 (Washington: U.S. Government Printing Office, 1973).

5. J. A. Curran, "Provision of Better Medical Care," *Milbank Memorial Fund Quarterly* 23 (1945): 7.

6. F. Jenson, H. G. Weiskotten, and M. S. Thomas, *Medical Care of the Discharged Hospital Patient* (New York: Commonwealth Fund, 1944).

7. M. D. Bogdonoff, S. W. Elwell, and J. Reffris, "Medical Outpatient Department Teaching," *Journal of Medical Education* 35 (1963): 885–89.

8. J. D. Rising, "The Rural Preceptorship," *Journal of the Kansas Medical Society* 63 (1962): 81–84.

9. J. H. Bakst, "A Domicilliary Care Program as an Integrated Facility in the Medical Curriculum," *Journal of the Association of American Medical Colleges* 25 (1950): 406–14.

10. G. G. Reader, "Organization and Development of a Comprehensive Care Program," *American Journal of Public Health* 44 (1964): 760–65.

11. P. V. Lee, *Medical Schools and the Changing Times* (Evanston, Illinois: Association of American Medical Colleges, 1962).

12. K. R. Hammond and F. Kern, *Teaching Comprehensive Medical Care: A Psychological Study of Change in Medical Education* (Cambridge: Harvard University Press, 1959).

13. G. G. Reader and M. E. Goss, *Comprehensive Medical Care and Teaching* (Ithaca: Cornell University Press, 1967).

14. J. H. Kennell, "Experience with a Medical School Family Health Study," *Journal of Medical Education* 36 (1961): 1649–1716.

15. J. J. Alpert, "Educating the Physician Towards a Solution," *Archives of Internal Medicine* 127 (1970): 85–88.

16. J. Millis, *Report of the Citizens Commission of Graduate Medical Education* (Chicago: American Medical Association, 1966).

17. S. A. Schroeder, S. M. Werner and T. E. Piemme, "Primary Care in the Academic Medical Centers: A Report of a Survey by the AAMC," *Journal of Medical Education* 49 (1974): 823–33.

18. D. H. Funkenstein, "Medical Students, Medical School and Society During Three Eras" in *Psychosocial Aspects of Medical Training*, ed. R. Coombs and C. Vincent (Springfield, Illinois: Charles C. Thomas, 1971).

DISCUSSION

One participant observed that the goals expressed by Alpert might be more readily achieved if it were admitted that most medical schools are not good enough to have such programs.

The Congress has confused the issues of primary care and geographic distribution. Distribution might be greatly benefited by a program to persuade the spouses of physicians of the advantages of relocation. Another problem is the use of the term "remote site," which to an urban dweller has a somewhat ominous ring, but which does not necessarily mean geographically remote.

With regard to the distribution and career choices of black physicians, and the likelihood of their returning to the inner city, it was noted that, after filtering out the graduates of Howard and Meharry medical schools, their pattern is the same as for white graduates.

In response to the observation that many Canadian schools have popular primary care programs in which the role of the community hospital is important, Alpert stated that community hospitals in the United States are not staffed by primary care physicians. In terms of decrease in the number of such physicians, the Canadian situation had not deteriorated as dramatically as it has in this country.

Turning to the role of nurse practitioners and physician's assistants, it was noted that although many perform the same functions as physicians, they are paid much less. A counter argument was that "jumping on the physician's assistants bandwagon" is easy, but it may serve only to preserve the status quo. While there is great respect for the skills and dedication of other health professionals, and recognition of the value of the primary care team, it was felt that the physician should retain final decision-making responsibility.

New Directions in Medical Education:
Family Medicine

EUGENE S. FARLEY, JR.

Family medicine enjoys the excitement and challenge of being a new specialty with clearly defined goals and responsibilities. The specialty arose in response to the recognized need of individuals and society for easier access to high-quality, integrated medical and health care. Since it draws on the knowledge and competencies of many other specialties, family medicine depends heavily on the integration of old, and the synthesis of new, knowledge to create its own identity and meet the needs of society and the individual patient.

From 1915 to 1965 internal medicine responded to pressures from society for increased knowledge of disease, better trained doctors, and quality care. The very success of internal medicine in these areas led to a narrowing of its focus and responsibilities until it was no longer responsive to society's health care needs. Family medicine is responding to a need and a demand, at all levels of society, for accessibility to high-caliber medical care. This care should be provided by well-trained physicians interested in providing it to all persons regardless of age, sex, or dis-ease.

DEFINITIONS

Family Practice

• Serves patients regardless of age, sex, or dis-ease (organic, psychological, or social).

• Is at risk to the patient with an undefined problem. The doctor must identify the problem and respond to it appropriately by: a) providing the care himself; b) referral to or consultation with others; or c) mobilization of needed resources.

180

- Provides continuity of care to the individual and the family. Its practitioners are obliged to respond to the evolution of health and dis-ease in an individual, family, and community.
- Deals with the individual in the context of the family and community. The practitioner's rewards come from dealing with the individual. The dis-ease is seen in the context of the patient. This is important if one is to avoid the concept of "crockism," or the patient having the "wrong" dis-ease for the interest of the doctor.
- Exposes its practitioners to the family and its problems as well as to the individual and his or her problems—potentially, therefore, he serves the whole family.
- Serves a community of patients.
- Cares for the common problems, whether simple or complex, including otitie medida, hypertension, depression, diabetes, lacerations, growth and development, and family problems.
- Identifies or appropriately suspects the uncommon problems and makes sure they receive appropriate attention. These may include leukemia, pheochromocytoma, hypopituitarism, and any other disorder the practitioner sees too rarely to maintain competence in.

Family Medicine

- Is the academic discipline that looks at and studies families and family practice; educates and trains students, residents, and practitioners in the concepts and tools needed in family practice; and develops new knowledge regarding family practice and family medicine.
- Has its roots in:

   General practice, which emphasizes provision of care to a population regardless of age, sex, or disease; access to care for the as yet undifferentiated problem; and access to the entire family.
   Pediatrics, which emphasizes growth and development; prevention through immunizations, guidance, and counseling; and the importance of the family and family relationships in child rearing and adolescence.
   Preventive, community, and/or social medicine, which emphasize outreach; community-wide prevention; early detection, and screening; and community, environmental, and social factors in disease.
   Internal medicine, which emphasizes knowledge of disease; clinical competence and skill; and the development of new knowledge.

Psychiatry, which emphasizes listening with the "third ear"; individual counseling and psychodynamics; family interactions and psychodynamics; and the treatment of emotional problems.

Social work, which emphasizes knowledge and use of community resources; and counseling the individual and the family.

Behavioral sciences (sociology, anthropology, psychology), which emphasize community structure and interactions; and family structures and relationships.

GENERAL PHILOSOPHICAL STATEMENTS
RELATING TO ALL HEALTH CARE

These statements are not unique to family medicine or family practice. They are, however, ideas and concepts that must be recognized by all those in family medicine and incorporated into the actions of those in family practice.

1. Health is the being in harmony with his environment. This definition integrates the organic, psychological, and social aspects of health and illness and avoids any prejudicial implications frequently found in other definitions. The danger is that it requires one to recognize or define the environment. If the immediate environment in which one lives is sick, and one is in harmony with it, that harmony may reflect illness in that individual. The practitioner must therefore be aware of the environment and develop some concepts as to its basic health. This latter is difficult but important, as all practitioners must be aware of the environment and develop some concepts as to its basic health. All practitioners must view the patient in the "context of his family and community."

2. The quality of secondary and tertiary care given is directly related to the quality of primary care. If there is limited access to appropriate primary care, the secondary and tertiary care specialists become inundated with the "wrong problems," in which by definition they are not interested, or, by training, prefer not to see in large numbers. If they must see too many "wrong problems" they quickly lose their skills in caring for the "right problems." The converse is also true. If there are too few or poorly trained secondary and tertiary care specialists, primary care specialists are forced to spend inordinate amounts of time on the rare or uncommon problems, and are then unavailable to care for the common ones. The health care of a population and the satisfaction of health

care providers is absolutely dependent on a proper mix of specialists in primary, secondary, and tertiary care.

3. All medical and health care is based on the patient's, family's, and/or community's strengths. For example, the patient with an acute myorcardial infarction survives because of the strength of the remaining functioning heart muscle; the patient with severe psychological disturbance functions at a level determined by his psychological reserves (strengths). All medical and health care must therefore develop around and build on these strengths: their idenfication is essential for the survival of the patient and for the psychological survival of the primary care doctor, as it is the patient's strengths which make him likeable as a person, even though it is his dis-ease (weakness) that brought him to the doctor.

4. Each doctor-patient contact must help reinforce the patient's strengths. This is important in order to prevent the patient, who is already in a dependent role, from relying excessively or chronically on that role. It is essential to help patients (all people) feel good about themselves in a realistic way so they can further develop their strengths and mobilize new ones to better handle the problems with which they are confronted.

Part of the helping-healing role of the provider is to help the patient "love himself" so he can better "love others," and, as a result, be "loved" by others and "grow" from this.

5. The doctor is a participating observer. He is asked by the patient to observe and identify the problems and then participate in their resolution by modification of behavior, whether organic (physical, chemical); psychological; or social or environmental.

6. One-upmanship is detrimental to sound learning and quality care. In medical education it encourages a doctor to hide his ignorance and limitations. Since quality is dependent on the provider fully recognizing the limits of his capabilities, and responding appropriately to these limits, it is important that he openly be encouraged to recognize and handle them in a supportive educational setting.

7. The doctor serves as the patient's entrée into the medical care system; the patient serves as the doctor's entrée into his family and community. The clinical and personal skills (real or imagined) of the doctor bring the patient to him with his dis-ease. The doctor must then use his skills to help the patient with his presenting problem and identify other potentially serious problems as they relate to the patient, his family, or community.

8. The patient care responsibilities of the primary physician expose him to the problems of mankind—individual, family, and community—and should make him socially aware.

9. Basic to all science and patient care are data collection; data organization; data analysis; and decision making.

10. Quantity and quality are inextricably related. If a community has fifty persons who need care and only thirty can get it, perhaps the community is receiving poor care; if fifty receive care with inadequate resources, the community may also be getting poor care. Quantity and quality must therefore be related if we are to serve communities. Response to this usually involves the use of additional health care providers.

11. All areas of medical education and research need a laboratory, whether it be a traditional research laboratory; the hospital; a practice; or the community.

RESPONSIBILITIES OF FAMILY MEDICINE IN GRADUATE EDUCATION

Graduate education in family medicine will be discussed before undergraduate education, because without the former, with its residents and faculty caring for patients, it can be difficult to teach family medicine adequately.

Family medicine must incorporate the above concepts into its teaching, while assuring:

1. Clinical competence, to allow identification and treatment of common problems; identification and referral (or securing consultations) for rare problems; prevention and screening when possible.

This requires use of the teaching and inpatient training capabilities of the traditional specialists. It also requires use of family practitioners and behavioral scientists in the model practice to help students and trainees use the knowledge acquired from the specialties rationally, in order to provide continuing comprehensive care and make appropriate sequential decisions during the evolution of health and dis-ease in the patient, family, and population served.

2. Awareness of individual and family psychodynamics, to provide the ability to intervene in early common problems and help relieve chronic problems; listen with the third ear, so as to appropriately identify and respond to indirect cues the patient may give regarding the problems; respond to the problem presented by the patient and identify other problems that may also need or respond to appropriate intervention; and deal with normal and stressed inter-

personal relationships, and, where possible, facilitate reduction of excess or pathological stress.

3. Awareness of cultural and social differences and community and societal dynamics affecting patients and patient care, to allow recognition of the difference between pathological or widely deviant behavior and culturally accepted or determined variations—this is necessary if the doctor is to clearly understand areas where behavior needs to be modified and where it does not; and recognition by the doctor that he, as the provider, is not the determiner or "model" for "normal" among the patients he serves.

4. Ability to use other health care providers, and recognition of how they work in the system. This must be done in a setting where the doctors and other health care providers can learn to work well together and use each other's skills appropriately. (The other providers include nurses, nurse practitioners, physician's associates, and social workers.)

5. Constant input from family practitioners, since family medicine is the academic discipline relating to family practice, which must include data from family practices.

6. Familiarity with data organization and use. Since family practice is a pragmatic approach to the application of knowledge and clinical skills to the health needs of a population, the data systems it incorporates and uses must be of value in practice—patient care and management; teaching—content, audit, and review: and research—prospective and retrospective, health care, and clinical.

These systems must allow us to look at individuals and populations, since that is the reality faced by practitioners of family medicine. The organization of the data collected must allow definition of the population served by the following parameters, at least: age and sex; dis-ease or problem; area of residence; family; individual; and socioeconomic background.

Data so organized is only of value if those collecting it are effective and trained observers. It is necessary for family medicine to teach future family practitioners the systems that allow this organization of data. It is important that these systems be simple so they faciliate, rather than interfere with, the provision of patient care.

SETTING IN WHICH TEACHING AND RESEARCH TAKE PLACE

To accomplish its educational goals, family medicine must have a laboratory and teaching setting, just as any other discipline. Traditional medical education in the clinical and postgraduate years uses the hospital as its laboratory and classroom. Family medicine deals with a community of patients at all levels of health and illness, and therefore more with the vertical than the horizontal patient. This means it must focus much of its teaching and most of its laboratory work in the practice and in the community.

Practice, rather than clinic, is intentionally used here, because *practice* implies an integrated system that controls the charts, the associated providers, such as nurses and nurse practitioners, and the secretaries. Practice is developed specifically to serve the needs and teach the care of the ambulatory patient, regardless of age, sex, or dis-ease, and places emphasis on continuity and comprehensiveness. *Clinic* frequently denotes that place in the hospital where patients are seen by providers who want to be elsewhere and who have no control or say as to the systems or methods used in providing care. The manner of care and systems used often assure discontinuous and episodic care, with little or no access to the family or community. This is often associated with precepting by faculty who also do not know the patient or community.

Family medicine practice laboratories are of two types:

1. Those controlled by the teaching program and its full-time faculty; and

2. Those controlled by full-time, practicing family practitioners who may be identified as community faculty.

The practice controlled by the teaching program provides: a) a population or community of patients that can be studied, as the faculty, trainees (residents), and students are responsible for its care: this facilitates clinical training and development and implementation of agreed-upon standards of care; b) the ability to study some aspects of health care and its provision through use of systems of data organization; identification of problems in the population served and in the systems used; and application of new systems or solutions that may be developed; c) clinical material to assure that doctors training in that setting have adequate experience and supervision to develop clinical competence; know how to care for a population of patients over a prolonged period; and be effective in making appropriate sequential decisions necessary in providing this care; and d) organized data systems.

Practices controlled by full-time practitioners provide a more efficient model and a more "real" practice situation. They also allow populations and problems seen in a purely teaching practice to be compared with those seen in purely service practices.

In the teaching practice, data organization systems must be in use, and there must be clear and easy access to the charts and control of them by those who provide care and who are responsible for teaching. Continuity of care must be built-in, with total coverage for the patients. There must be immediate preception available by "faculty" experienced in ambulatory care and community practice. The practice must serve whole families as well as segments of families. Students must be aware of the role of the family, care for the whole family, and yet be able to care for any member who may leave it and yet still wants treatment. In this setting the student must be supervised and precepted in family and individual counseling, so he becomes comfortable with family psychodynamics and to working with the entire family.

In this practice the common problems must be emphasized, whether simple or complex, so the student or trainee is able to recognize, treat, and, when possible, prevent them. Dealing with a reasonably diverse practice population will assure the presence of less common problems, which must be identified and appropriately handled by referral or consultation. In the teaching setting, additional consultations will be obtained for their educational and teaching value so the trainee can learn to handle and care for them. Knowledge of the latest treatment or of the pathophysiology of uncommon problems does not need emphasis in family practice. If one is identified, and the family doctor plans or needs to be involved in its continuing care and treatment, he must then learn more about it.

The proper data organization system is essential if the practice is to serve as a laboratory from which old knowledge is studied and new knowledge developed. Such organization provides the capability to record and retrieve data collected in caring for a patient. It can facilitate the provision of comprehensive and continuous care, and allow identification of what has and has not been done in providing care. Such systems allow study of the patient population served and identification of its problems. They facilitate patient care; appropriate use of resources; outreach; application of new knowledge; self- and continuing medical education; audit; and identification of new knowledge and problems.

Data organization identifies:

1. The individual as represented by the chart, which should have a structure and defined data base; flow sheets; and problem sheet and problem-oriented notes.

2. The family, which can be represented by the folder—charts of all members of the family (or household) can be filed in the same folder, or under the family number.

3. The practice, which can be represented by: a) the age-sex register: each male interviewed has a blue card filled out with his name, address, and date of birth, which is filed under year of birth; for each female the same is done with a pink card—this quickly provides a running count of the practice population by age and sex, and can then be compared with the population characteristics of the whole community; and b) the problem or diagnostic index, which requires coding of the problems identified in the patient population and allows retrieval of all individuals in the practice with the problems coded; the index allows studies of cohorts of patients by problem or disease, and facilitates review, outreach, audit, and application of new knowledge to patients with the identified problem.

4. The community, which can be represented by the method of filing: geographic filing, or filing by census tracts allows all those who live near each other to be filed together; it is simplified by color-coding the family or household folder by area of residence. This allows easy relation of census bureau sociodemographic information of specific census tracts to the population served from that tract. It also permits problems seen in the practice to be related to geographic areas and/or population groups.

Since family medicine deals with populations as well as with the individual and family, it has incorporated the above concepts into its teaching practice model. Although these systems are not unique to family medicine, at the present time it is the only specialty involved in medical education that feels it important to teach practical, practice-oriented, data organization systems. To assure their use in practice they must be taught before a physician enters practice, so their use, problems, and potential are understood. Ideally the teaching of these or compatible systems should occur in undergraduate medical education.

PROPOSALS FOR INTEGRATING FAMILY MEDICINE INTO THE UNDERGRADUATE MEDICAL CURRICULUM

Family medicine is unique among the specialties in that it is truly interdisciplinary or cross-disciplinary, and must therefore have the cooperation of other departments. Since its goals and responsibilities differ from these departments, however, its acceptance by them is often limited. They may feel threatened by it, perceiving it as infringing on their areas of competence or responsibility, or on their resources, or as training doctors in a different way than they do. They may disagree with family medicine's basic concepts, or dismiss them without considering them.

As a result of its interdisciplinary nature, the areas of undergraduate education with which family medicine is involved vary from school to school. In some, it may assume responsibility for teaching in the areas of the doctor-patient relationship; interviewing and history taking; physical examination and diagnosis; or community resources and outreach. In others, these areas may already be adequately covered by other departments or faculty. In all schools it must teach in those areas unique to family medicine, which include access to and care of families and populations of patients.

In most medical schools family medicine is unique in that it has its own group of patients for whose ongoing care it is responsible. It is these patients and the setting in which they receive care (the practice) to which students must be exposed.

1. *Early clinical experience.* This should not be done as a random, uncontrolled experience with poorly defined goals, but as a well-planned, controlled experience with goals appropriate to the level of the student. These goals can be graded so that the student: a) works with practice nurses to learn to do TPR, BP, height and weight, etc.; take a simple didactic history by filling out base-line history forms on each patient seen; and do simple routine office laboratory procedures such as hematocrits, urinalysis, and blood counts; b) learns from doctors, nurse practitioners, and physician's assistants how to be comfortable with the patient and with themselves at each stage of learning, so they can better understand the fine points offered in subsequent stages of learning, and function at their level of competence; and c) learns how to recognize common physical findings and variations, normal and abnormal.

Students should always be identified and introduced as such in order that they may feel at ease with the patient at their own level of knowledge, and not have to "bluff" through a situation as "doctor." This is extremely important, and the teacher must, in front of the patient, help students to recognize and be comfortable with their limitations. The teacher must not teach or reinforce the development of evasive strategies. In practice the doctor must always be aware of and recognize his limitations, and acceptance of this fact must be taught and reinforced.

2. *Data organization.* Each student can and should keep an age-sex registry and diagnostic index on all the patients he sees or learns from. Ideally these should be kept through all four years of medical school, with periodic audit by the faculty to be sure the students are seeing an adequate number and variety of problems appropriate for the training of the undifferentiated physician or for the specialty they may later be entering.

These systems facilitate student review of the problems or patients they have seen. They allow the students to look at cohorts of patients and populations to better relate to the practice of medicine some of the concepts and methodologies learned in preventive medicine. Students can learn to apply practical epidemiology to the community of patients seen in their training and by doctors in practice. Precepting can be facilitated as the preceptor and student together review the problems seen by the students and thereby identify experience and shortcomings in knowledge and/or skill that need to be corrected.

3. *Psychodynamics of patients and families,* "normal" and "abnormal." This can be most valuable when done in conjunction with family doctors, psychiatrists, psychologists, and others who are able to help the student pick out and recognize the unidentified or undefined emotional problem. This gives the student an exposure to and awareness of family issues and problems not usually seen by psychiatrists, social workers, and psychologists, as well as of those commonly seen by these specialists.

In the setting of the family practice, and with responsibility for the care of the whole family, the student can learn about the developmental stages of the family and the concept of family life cycles, which are important to understanding the stresses of the individual coming from that family.

Family medicine must put a great deal of emphasis on its integrative teaching if the foregoing concepts are to be used in the daily function and practice of those it trains.

Synthesis of new knowledge is an important part of the practicality and excitement of medicine. In family medicine the integration and synthesis may largely be from data (observations) obtained in the care of patients and populations, and should include:

- The natural history of disease;
- Family evolution and development; and
- Studies of individuals, families, populations, and care systems, in general, including medical and health care systems, large or small.

THE FUTURE

Family medicine as an academic discipline and as a service discipline faces many obstacles. These come from:

1. *Traditional academia*—those who know the answers; those who deny the issues or refuse to look at them; those who think it is a passing fad; and those who believe family medicine has no goals or knowledge base, because they have looked at one incompletely developed program and found it inadequate, or have not differentiated between family medicine and general practice.

Traditional academicians have often thought that anyone could do primary care; that there is nothing unique or special about it; that it is not challenging; that it is not fun; that it deals only with colds and runny noses; and that no one would want to do it if he had a choice.

2. *Methods of financing graduate medical education.* Traditional graduate medical education was developed to meet the care needs of hospitalized patients, and as a result has been supported from inpatient-care dollars. As yet there are no secure sources of funding for the training of doctors in primary care. Although it brings in the fewest dollars per unit of care of any of the specialties, particularly the procedure-oriented specialties, it requires concentration of teaching resources around that unit of care. Primary care education is therefore the least apt to ever be self-supporting from the patient-care dollar.

Since family medicine's major responsibility is the training of primary care doctors, it has limited access to hospital funds. Internal medicine and pediatrics, with strong roots in the hospital and hospital funding, have primarily inpatient responsibilities and are therefore not as free to develop fully their primary care training potential; at the same time they are much more secure in their long-term funding. The pressures for inpatient care and funding from this care, plus the need to train many different types of subspecialists, diffuse their responsibility for primary training and provide them with little need or incentive to change this responsibility significantly.

If the medical education system, undergraduate and graduate, is rational, it will look further at its responsibilities for training primary care doctors, study methods of funding this training, and recognize that no one group has answered, to anyone's satisfaction, the problems of primary care for all our citizens. It will recognize that family medicine can only develop and contribute if the system, with leadership from hospital administrators, departmental chairmen, and medical school deans, is willing to support it and reallocate resources. This latter is hard for well-established medical schools and residency programs to accept, as they have been succeeding very well in what they have been doing and may not consider this new role—training doctors to meet the needs of the health care system—as one they want or need.

For family medicine to develop in hospitals and medical schools, the deans and faculty will have to recognize and support the necessity for an interdepartmental approach. Strong leadership in the specialty will be needed to assure its goals in education are met and not confused or hidden by the goals of other departments that participate in training family doctors. Since, in reality, family medicine attempts to achieve the best that educators talk about in a broadly trained doctor with experience and training across the disciplines, it seems that barriers to its development should be lowered. Family medicine can contribute to other disciplines as they attempt to develop their primary care training programs, just as they contribute to the education of family doctors in the inpatient setting and in some of the specialty clinics.

We hope the medical education system will study its responsibility and respond to the need to train doctors appropriately for the system in which most of them will work, as well as for the needs of the society they are to serve.

DISCUSSION

One reason few students enter family practice is that they are not exposed to it in medical school. Many schools have only a handful of family practice faculty members, and the students who come into contact with them are already oriented to the field.

Another reason for the reluctance of students to become family practitioners is a fear of appearing incompetent. Many feel it is safer to specialize in just one area. Yet what impresses students who are exposed to family practice programs is working with a group of doctors who are not afraid to say, "I don't know."

A priority should be the establishment of better communication between the medical center and the family doctor. It was suggested that medical centers should set up a central office that the family doctor who needs advice on a problem could contact for referral to the appropriate faculty member.

The identification of an academic base for family medicine is a problem. Without such a base, family medicine may not flourish as an academic discipline.

Regional Medical Education: The WAMI Program

M. ROY SCHWARTZ

PACIFIC NORTHWEST AND ALASKA

There are, in the Pacific Northwest and Alaska, four states referred to as "WAMI territory"—*W*ashington, *A*laska, *M*ontana and *I*daho, from which the acronym WAMI was taken. These states collectively represent 22 percent of the land mass of the United States, cover five time zones, and have cities separated by distances exceeding that between Los Angeles and New York City. As an example of the immensity of the area, when the tide recedes in the state of Alaska, more land is recovered than exists in the entire state of Texas. It is therefore not surprising that enormous geographic barriers must be surmounted in any effort concerned with regionalized medical education or health care in the WAMI territory.

While the WAMI territory offers a variety of options for living styles and recreation, it also has some serious problems:

1. The University of Washington School of Medicine in Seattle is the only medical school in the four-state area. Moreover, Alaska, Montana, and Idaho are financially unable to build and operate schools of their own, and Washington cannot support a second medical school even though the population of the state would justify one.

2. In the past five years the expansion in the pool of applicants to medical schools in the United States has been so great that two to three qualified applicants are now being rejected for each one accepted. As a consequence, there has been growing pressure on state-supported medical schools, such as that of the University of Washington, to limit enrollment to residents of the supporting state and to discriminate against those from states without medical schools, such as Alaska, Montana, and Idaho.

194

Moreover, in the area of graduate medical education there is a limited number of available training posts in the Pacific Northwest and Alaska. Since between 50 and 70 percent of those physicians who take their graduate training in a given area remain there to practice, this limitation has enormous significance for the WAMI states.

Finally, because of the geographic and communications barriers in the WAMI territory, only a limited number of options are available for the continuing medical education of practicing physicians. This deficiency is especially critical in rural areas of the four states that constitute the greater part of the WAMI territory.

3. In addition to the needs in health education, the WAMI region has vexing and challenging health care problems. In the first place there are not enough primary care physicians, and those who are in practice are clustered around the major metropolitan centers. As a consequence, the extensive rural areas have an insufficient number of primary care physicians. This, coupled with the progressive trend toward early retirement for physicians, has led to an inadequate pool of manpower, which is not distributed according to population needs. There is thus great variation in the health services available to residents of the WAMI states.

THE WAMI PROGRAM

In 1968 the University of Washington School of Medicine responded to these problems by modifying its undergraduate medical education curriculum. In its new curriculum, time was made the variable and achievement the constant, so that students could graduate in as little as three years or as long as six years. Exposure to clinical medicine was initiated in the first year of undergraduate education, and approximately 40 percent of the curriculum time was made elective in order to provide for flexibility of career training. Included among these options was a new family medicine pathway designed to attract and train students in the area of primary care.

The new curriculum also set the stage for the development of the WAMI experiment in decentralized medical education. Conceived in December 1969, it had five goals:

1. Increase the number of students admitted from the WAMI states;

2. Increase the number of primary care physicians being trained;

3. Bring the resources of the medical center to communities in the WAMI territory;

4. Accomplish the programmatic goals without the requirement of new "bricks and mortar," or capital building, programs; and

5. Place physicians in areas of need, or redress the maldistribution of physicians that exists in the region.

To accomplish these goals a two-phase program was implemented in March 1971. The objectives of the first, or *university phase,* was to present the first year of undergraduate medical education at four universities without medical schools in the WAMI states: the University of Alaska in Fairbanks; Montana State University in Bozeman; Washington State University in Pullman; and the University of Idaho in Moscow. Upon completion of their first year, students enroll at the School of Medicine in Seattle, where they take their second year of training and most of their third. When they have finished the introductory clerkships in internal medicine, pediatrics, obstetrics and gynecology, surgery, and psychiatry, the students are offered the option of participating in the *community phase* of the program.

The objective of the community phase is to provide undergraduate students and residents in graduate medical education with structured community-based clerkship experiences in the rural or "need" areas of the WAMI states. To achieve this, practicing physicians in selected communities have been given clinical appointments in the School of Medicine and are remunerated for their time. Students and residents are sent to these communities for six weeks to six months of formal clinical training. The sponsoring department selects the community, and is responsible for all training. While there, students not only diagnose and treat disease, but gain a perspective of the roles of, challenges to, and demands on a practicing physician in such a setting. It is anticipated that such exposure will encourage students and residents to settle in similar communities to practice.

In order to monitor the program, faculty from the School of Medicine visit these "community clinical units" every six weeks to assess the academic progress of the students and residents, to provide input to their training, and to give consultative assistance to physicians and other health professionals in the area. In this way the continuing medical education resources of the medical center are brought to the community level in an attempt to keep these health professionals abreast of new knowledge and skills.

At the present time the WAMI program operates fourteen community clinical units, as follows:

1. *Family Medicine.* Alaska: Kodiak; Washington: Omak, Grandview, Anacortes, and Whidbey Island; Montana: Whitefish-Kalispell;

2. *Pediatrics.* Idaho: Pocatello; Montana: Great Falls; Washington: Spokane;

3. *Internal Medicine.* Montana: Billings and Missoula; Washington: Wenatchee;

4. *Obstetrics and Gynecology.* Idaho: Boise;

5. *Psychiatry.* Alaska: Anchorage.

ATS-6 COMMUNICATIONS SATELLITE EXPERIMENTS

Two challenges continue to pose problems for components of the WAMI program. These include the need for communication between participants in the educational program, and the need to monitor the quality of the educational experience. Hence it has been necessary to define ways in which a unique resource located in Seattle, such as an endocrinologist, can be shared with institutions and communities that lack this expertise but require it for curricular purposes.

For this reason the School of Medicine was intrigued by the possibilities that two-way, interactive, full-duplex video and full-duplex audio communications might offer in meeting these challenges, and undertook a series of experiments via the ATS-6 satellite to explore their advantages. The experiments were conducted between Seattle and Fairbanks, and between Seattle and Omak, a rural town in the north central part of Washington.

In the experiment between Seattle and Fairbanks, it was found that communication in full-duplex video and audio was feasible; only half-duplex video and full-duplex audio were available between Seattle and Omak. In addition, a color video signal was transmitted between Seattle and Fairbanks; the image signal between Seattle and Omak was totally in black-and-white, except for a small number of broadcasts done in color for experimental and comparison purposes.

From September 1974 through May 1975 the following experiments were carried out:

1. *Student Affairs.* Admissions interviews were held in which some members of the Admissions Committee were located in Seattle,

while the candidates and the remaining members of the committee were located in Fairbanks. In addition to the interviews, student advising, counseling, and orientation services were provided, with the advisor or counselor in Seattle and the students in Fairbanks.

2. *Curriculum: University Phase.* In the university phase of the curricular experiments, lectures, small group discussions, and laboratory and clinical demonstrations were transmitted from Seattle to Fairbanks and vice versa.

3. *Curriculum: Community Phase.* In the community phase, students presented their cases (patients) to their mentors in Seattle, who in turn assessed the skill with which the students had performed the patient work-up and the knowledge they had acquired about the patient. The mentors offered assistance in evaluating the particular problem at hand, and in this way contributed to the students' education. In addition, discussions of problem cases were held between faculty in Omak and in Seattle. Finally, continuing education was conducted via specialty conferences in such disciplines as radiology, psychiatric counseling, and general internal medicine.

4. *Health Care.* In the area of health care delivery, a series of consultations were held between dermatologists in Seattle and patients in Fairbanks. In these experiments a dermatologist viewed a patient, proposed a diagnosis to a local practicing physician, and suggested a course of therapy. Discussions and consultations were also provided in radiology, rehabilitation medicine, and psychiatry.

5. *Evaluations.* In terms of students' performances, a series of experimental evaluations were made, including oral and laboratory examinations. In addition, students were allowed access via the satellite to the computer-aided evaluation (CAE) data banks located at Ohio State University. In this experiment the link between the terminals in Fairbanks and Seattle was made via the ATS-6 satellite, and the computer at Ohio State was linked to Seattle via telephone ground line. This experiment was designed to determine to what extent the independent study program, which has been in existence at the University of Washington School of Medicine for four years, could, with its attendant computer-aided instruction and evaluation modules, be transplanted to a university without presenting the entire program.

6. *Administration.* In the administrative arena, a series of conferences were held with the participation of faculty, students, and administrators. The purpose was to plan, work out differences of opinion, analyze budgets, and evaluate the progress of the program.

LESSONS LEARNED AND CONCLUSIONS DRAWN

While a variety of conclusions may be drawn from the experiments conducted via the ATS-6 satellite, only five will be discussed here:

1. Both video and audio interactions are a necessary prerequisite for successful transmission of admissions interviews, counseling sessions, administrative conferences, laboratory and clinical demonstrations, small group discussions, case presentations, and health care delivery experiments.

2. Color video adds a necessary dimension to some of the experiments, but it was especially critical for the dermatology consultations, clinical and laboratory demonstrations, laboratory evaluations, and in some cases psychiatric counseling.

3. It is possible to conduct a major educational program and provide health care via interactive communications satellite, and thereby share resources and avoid travel. This is particularly true of those components of education and health care delivery that require video signals.

4. None of the satellite experiments were, however, any better than the "software" preparation that preceded the broadcasts. It became apparent that an enormous amount of software preparation was necessary in order to produce effective programs that could be evaluated in an appropriate manner. It is our opinion that without an investment in software, the experiments should not be conducted.

5. Interactive video and audio have broad applicability, and hence will play a major role in both health education and the provision of health care in the future. With this telecommunications link it should be possible to avoid the necessity of building three or four new medical schools in the WAMI territory, and at the same time accomplish the programmatic goals of communication between the component parts and evaluate the educational experiences in the WAMI undertaking. Since the satellite does not respect time or geographic and political boundaries, its applicability seems almost limitless.

RESULTS TO DATE

So far the results of the WAMI program in relation to the five programmatic objectives are as follows:

- *Objective.* To increase the number of students admitted to medical school from the WAMI states.

Developments:

As may be seen in Table 1, the enrollment of students from all WAMI states has expanded in the five years the WAMI program has been in operation, compared to the previous five years. The most dramatic increases have been in the AMI states, where only small numbers of students were admitted to the University of Washington School of Medicine in the five years before the WAMI program was initiated. Objective number one has therefore been achieved.

• *Objective.* To increase the numbers of primary care physicians being trained.

Developments:

Since the advent of the WAMI program there has been a significant increase in the number of students choosing the family medicine pathway (Table 2). When the number who participated in the university phase of the program was compared to non-WAMI participants, relative to choice of a curricular pathway, it was discovered that program participants are choosing family medicine almost twice as frequently as their colleagues. In addition, some students who wish to pursue careers in primary care are selecting the clinical specialist pathway of the curriculum, and are taking training in other primary care disciplines such as internal medicine, pediatrics, and obstetrics and gynecology. These students have not, however, been clearly differentiated as choosing primary care, and, as such, are not identifiable at the present time. It appears from the data that this objective is being met.

• *Objective.* To bring the resources of the medical center to communities in the WAMI territory.

Developments:

Many approaches have been attempted to bring the resources of the

TABLE 1. NUMBER OF STUDENTS ADMITTED TO THE UNIVERSITY OF WASHINGTON SCHOOL OF MEDICINE

	Absolute Number		Average Number per Year		
State	Pre-WAMI 1965–70	Post-WAMI 1971–75	Pre-WAMI	Post-WAMI	Increase (Percent)
Washington	360	516	72.0	103.2	43
Alaska	3	30	0.6	6.0	900
Montana	7	42	1.4	8.4	500
Idaho	9	47	1.8	9.4	222

TABLE 2. NUMBER OF STUDENTS CHOOSING FAMILY MEDICINE
PATHWAY SINCE THE WAMI PROGRAM WAS INAUGURATED

Before WAMI	
1968–70	88
Since WAMI	
1971–73	147

medical center to the areas of need. Among these are visits of the
faculty to the universities and community clinical units: in the academic year 1974–75, twenty-eight faculty visits were made, during
which 1,439 physicians and health professionals attended courses or
teaching sessions. In this way they were made aware of the unique
health care resources available in Seattle. Among these resources are
centers for burns, neonatology, trauma, clinical research, and trans-
plants, and a regional cancer center. In addition, arrangements are
made for circuit courses to cities in the WAMI region; preceptorships
for physicians at the medical center; and short courses, seminars, and
sabbaticals.

• *Objective.* To accomplish programmatic goals without the requirement of new "bricks and mortar," or capital building, programs.
Developments:

To date, no new capital construction has occurred or is contemplated
as a result of the WAMI program. Minor remodeling has been or will
be done in a few locations.

• *Objective.* To place physicians in areas of need, or redress the
maldistribution that exists in the WAMI territory.
Developments:

The WAMI program has not been operating long enough to provide
a definitive answer to the question of whether it is meeting this goal.
The available data are found in Table 3, which shows the location of
residents who participated in the WAMI program and who are now in
practice. As may be seen, a sizable percentage of these graduates are
located in "rural" settings or in towns with populations of less than
five thousand. It remains to be seen whether this trend continues.
It should be pointed out that some physicians in the rural areas are
practicing in the National Health Service Corps, which has facilitated
their placement in rural communities.

In summary, four of the five objectives of the program have been
or are being met. While preliminary data is encouraging relative to
the last goal, insufficient information is available to warrant a

TABLE 3. LOCATION OF RESIDENTS WHO PARTICIPATED IN THE
WAMI PROGRAM

Type of Practice	Number	Percent
Rural	20	31.3
Inner city	2	3.1
Military	4	6.3
Faculty	1	1.6
Other	5	7.7
N.A.	3	4.7
In training	29	45.3

Note: Of the 35 who have completed their training, 57 percent have chosen rural practices.

definitive judgment as to whether the WAMI program has had an impact on the geographical maldistribution of physicians.

SUMMARY

This paper began with a discussion of the Pacific Northwest and Alaska, including the problems in health education and the provision of health care that exist in these regions of the United States. In addition, a review was made of the WAMI program and its efforts in the area of the continuum of medical education. Finally, the experiments conducted via the ATS-6 satellite were outlined, and the lessons and conclusion drawn from this series of experiments were discussed.

DISCUSSION

In response to a question, Schwartz said that no commitment is required of WAMI students to practice in the state. The medical school believes this to be unconstitutional—a form of indentured servitude.

The WAMI program is an example of remarkable organization and leadership. There are two key facets to the solution of the problem of geographic and specialty distribution: major efforts on the part of educational institutions, and regional considerations, that is, the identification of deficits and excesses in medical care in a given area. Regional resources, including educational progress such as WAMI, will be the basis for the resolution of the problem.

Regional Medical Education: The University of Illinois

WILLIAM J. GROVE

The purpose of this report is to describe the regionalized medical education program of the University of Illinois—its history, objectives, organization, curriculum, accomplishments, and problems. Even though each of these areas could be developed extensively and in great detail, this paper will merely provide an overview of the program.

The College of Medicine consists of a series of schools bound together as a collegium, in accordance with the statutes of the university. The regional program began to evolve more than a decade ago, with the very strong support of the president and executive vice president of the university. Inspired by the president, stimulated by the Center for Educational Development, a unit created in 1959 with the help of the Commonwealth Fund, and encouraged by a sympathetic chancellor and a forward-looking dean, the faculty had by 1963 developed a statement of goals that began: "The College of Medicine exists to promote improvement in the health of the public, and all its varied activities are so dedicated."

With the adoption of so broad a statement, the faculty, perhaps unknowingly, unfettered itself from viewing its roles as solely those of conducting research and educating physicians. Slowly it began to take a broader look at college responsibilities, addressing such issues as the shortage of physicians, at that time seen as particularly acute in rural areas of Illinois; continuing education; education of minorities; specialty training; and the provision of health care. The numerous published studies that discussed the social issues relating to health care needs were the "textbooks" for faculty study and planning.[1–8]

By 1967 the faculty had resolved to: 1) increase substantially the

203

production of physicians; 2) assume leadership in investigating with other colleges of the university various approaches to greater efficiency and productivity in the basic education of personnel for the health professions; and 3) assume leadership in studying the possibility of establishing additional affiliations in order to provide the clinical facilities necessary for expansion.

Subsequent to approval of these resolutions, a task force was appointed to develop plans for implementation of the broad objectives. It made eight recommendations, of which four are of continuing interest: 1) that the capability be developed to admit at least four hundred M.D. degree candidates annually by 1976; 2) that student attrition be balanced by admission to advanced standing; 3) that the growth be accommodated by creating semiautonomous schools of moderate size within the College of Medicine; and 4) that quality control of the educational programs continue to be exercised by the total faculty through a system of college committees responsible to an executive committee—later defined as the Academic Council.

At about the same time the medical faculty was developing its plans for growth, the Illinois Board of Higher Education, a coordinating agency for all of higher education, established a commission to make recommendations for further development of health professions within the state. The board mandated that the College of Medicine increase the number of graduates by at least two hundred as rapidly as possible, and augment its capability to teach one year of basic sciences. It urged the university to develop and expand additional clinical centers for the teaching of transitional and core clinical years, via affiliations with existing facilities in the Chicago metropolitan area, Peoria, and Rockford, and recommended that it investigate the potential of other clinical facilities for future medical education in Urbana–Champaign.

In September 1968 the faculty authorized the dean of the College of Medicine to appoint yet another group, which became known as the Committee to Coordinate Planning, to provide the final details for implementation of the expansion program. The committee was served by six subcommittees involving a wide spectrum of faculty and students. The report of that committee created the organization essentially as it is today. The plan was implemented on 1 January 1970.

ORGANIZATION

The University of Illinois was chartered in 1867, following the enactment in 1862 of the Morrill Land Grant College Act. At present the university consists of three major campuses. The largest is located in Urbana–Champaign, 128 miles south of Chicago; the other two are in close proximity, on Chicago's near west side: the Chicago Circle campus is just west of the Loop, or main business area of Chicago; the Medical Center campus is located one mile west of the Chicago Circle campus, in the midst of the 363-acre Medical Center district.

The university has five distinct administrative levels: 1) university or central administration, located predominantly on the Urbana–Champaign campus, headed by the chief executive officer, the president; 2) the campus level, with each of the three campuses being presided over by a chancellor; 3) the college level, served by a dean (with the exception of the College of Medicine, which has an executive dean); 4) the school level, where the presiding officer is called either a dean or director (in the College of Medicine the chief executive officers are called deans); and 5) the department, where the presiding officer is a head or chairman. The medical center campus (Figure 1) consists of the colleges of dentistry, pharmacy, nursing, graduate studies, public health, and medicine, and supporting services such as the library and biological resources laboratory.

The College of Medicine (Figure 2) consists of the Office of the Executive Dean, which includes the Center for Educational Development, the Area Health Education System, and offices of international and minority affairs; the School of Basic Medical Sciences, a one-year school located on the Medical Center campus; the School of Basic Medical Sciences, a one-year school located on the Urbana–Champaign campus; the Abraham Lincoln School of Medicine, which includes in its teaching resources a consortium of six metropolitan community hospitals; the Peoria School of Medicine, a three-year clinical school located in temporary quarters on the campus of Bradley University, 160 miles southwest of Chicago; the Rockford School of Medicine, a three-year clinical school located in an old tuberculosis sanitarium to which has been added a large wing for the library, auditorium, classrooms, offices, etc., eighty miles northwest of Chicago; and the School of Associated Medical Sciences, located on the Medical Center campus.

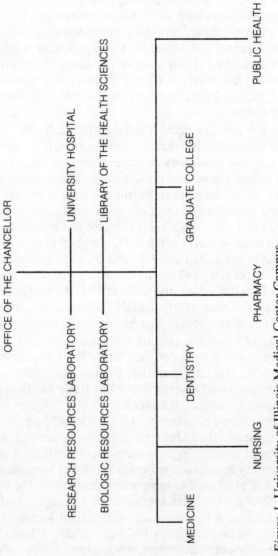

Figure 1. University of Illinois Medical Center Campus.

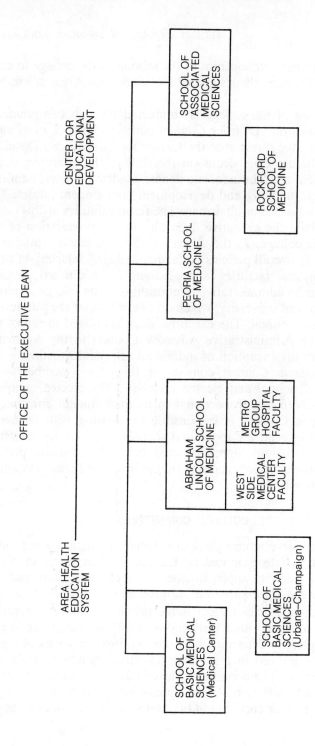

Figure 2. University of Illinois College of Medicine.

The geographic relationships of the schools of the college to each other and to the recently designated Health Service Areas are shown in Figure 3.

The business of the college is conducted through two councils. The *Administrative Advisory Council* consists of the dean of each of the schools, the director of the Center for Educational Development, and the associate deans on the staff of the executive dean. Currently there are four associate deans: academic affairs, administrative affairs, planning and development, and student affairs. The executive dean serves as chairman. The responsibilities of this council are to advise the executive dean on: 1) the preparation of the budget of the college; 2) the allocation of funds made available to the college; 3) overall policies on faculty and staff salaries; 4) utilization of physical facilities, and planning for additional physical facilities; and 5) administrative relationships of the college, external to the college and university, which do not fall under the purview of the Academic Council. The executive dean is obliged to report the actions of the Administrative Advisory Council to the Academic Council, with the exception of individual salary information.

The *Academic Council* consists of thirty-four members—the deans of each school and elected members. The elected members from each school are proportional to its total student enrollment. The Academic Council is responsible for dealing with academic issues that transcend the individual schools, with special reference to student admissions, appraisal, and promotion, faculty promotions, educational policy, and research policy. The faculty organization is shown in Figure 4.

COLLEGE COMMITTEES

The college level committees are elected annually by the entire faculty from a slate proposed by the college Committee on Committees. All students apply to one office of admissions and are admitted by the *Committee on Admissions*.

Prior academic achievement is the primary criterion for admission. As in so many other institutions, a faculty committee is currently struggling to determine how noncognitive attributes of candidates can be utilized in a manner objective enough to withstand judicial scrutiny. The committee has considered the idea of admission by random selection. At the time of acceptance, students state their preference for enrolling in the basic science school in Urbana–

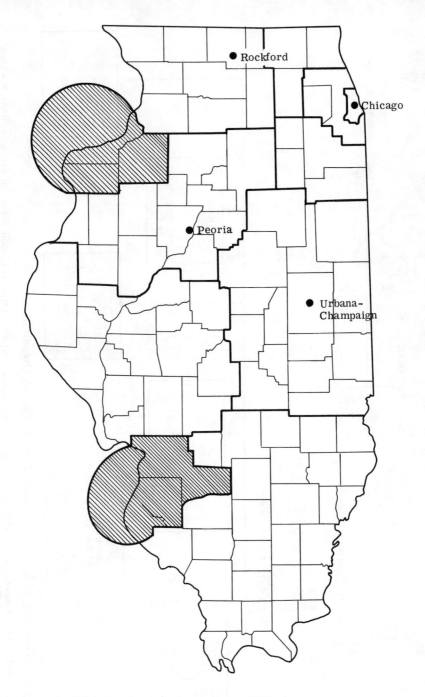

Figure 3. Health Service Areas in the State of Illinois.

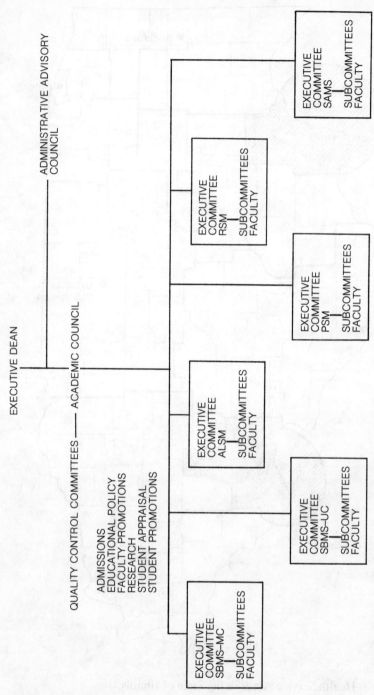

Figure 4. University of Illinois College of Medicine, Faculty Organization.

Code: SBMS–MC, School of Basic Medical Sciences, Medical Center; ALSM, Abraham Lincoln School of Medicine; RSM, Rockford School of Medicine; SBMS–UC, School of Basic Medical Sciences, Urbana–Champaign; PSM, Peoria School of Medicine; SAMS, School of Associated Medical Sciences.

Champaign or in the Medical Center campus in Chicago. In the fall of 1975, when 332 students were admitted, for example, 100 were accommodated in Urbana–Champaign and 232 in Chicago. At the time of acceptance, also, students are asked to express a preference for clinical schools in Chicago, Peoria, or Rockford. There has been no difficulty in matching requests and places in any of the schools.

Since 1970 the number of applicants to the College of Medicine has been proportional to the general increase in applicants throughout the United States. There were approximately twenty-eight hundred applicants for the class entering in 1975.

The *Committee on Student Appraisal* is responsible for administering the certifying examinations upon which a determination is made as to whether a student is qualified to move from a basic science school to a clinical school or is qualified to graduate. The committee, with staff support from the Center for Educational Development and participation of representatives of all disciplines and schools, prepares the certifying examinations. It has made extensive use of clinical simulation examinations [9] as a supplement to multiple-choice questions, and has selected test items according to the several levels of Bloom's taxonomy of educational objectives. National board examinations, Parts I and II are required, and, although technically possible, no student has been graduated who has not passed them, in addition to the internal certifying examination. Each school has an examination committee that prepares and administers noncertifying teaching or advisory examinations.

The *Committee on Student Promotions* receives reports of students' performances on the internal certifying examinations and the national board examinations from the Committee on Student Appraisal. The promotions committees of the schools provide the college promotion committee with information concerning each student's clinical performance and descriptions of consistent behavioral characteristics. It is the college committee that ultimately recommends those students who are to be promoted to the clinical schools from the basic science schools and those who are to be graduated. These recommendations are approved by the Academic Council. The college Committee on Student Promotions also serves as an appeal mechanism for students or faculty who believe that information provided by individual schools has been inaccurate or unfair.

Recommendations for tenured faculty appointments and promotions arise within departments of the schools, are approved within the schools by mechanisms designed by them, and are passed on to the college *Committee on Faculty Appointments, Promotions, and Tenure,* which makes final recommendations to the Academic Council.

The *Committee on Research* is responsible for reviewing and recommending action on all requests for research funds disbursed by the college. General research support grants have been, for the most part, controlled by the Committee on Research. Each of the schools is free to seek additional research funding independently. The committee is available to help new faculty members and new schools initiate research programs.

The *Committee on Educational Policy* is charged with responsibility to review the educational program of each school and to make recommendations to the Academic Council concerning curricula. This committee works through a series of ad hoc curriculum review committees that carry out a biennial peer review of each school's program. Every curriculum is based on objectives that have been carefully set down in documents of substantial size. In 1974 the College of Medicine faculty accepted corporate responsibility for graduate medical education. A subcommittee on graduate medical education has developed guidelines for review of these programs, the first two of which have now been approved by the Academic Council.

The Committee on Educational Policy has subcommittees on minority group affairs and on the independent study program. The efforts of the college to engage the issue of minorities in medicine has been described by Plagge and his colleagues; [10] Johns and Smith have reported the experiences of the faculty with an independent study program. [11]

CURRICULA

Since the 1950s the College of Medicine has endeavored to expand basic science learning experiences in the clinical years and to introduce more clinical medicine into the so-called basic science years. Clinical correlation clinics were tried in the first two basic science years, and basic science correlation conferences were offered in the clinical years; other schemes were also devised, but no actual integration has occurred. The literature suggests that such efforts at integration have been attempted in many schools.

When the college was reorganized into a series of schools, the preclinical portion of the curriculum was deliberately reduced to one year, during which the fundamental aspects of the basic sciences were to be learned. Clinically oriented basic sciences were to be extended throughout the three years of clinical instruction. With the exception of pathology and pharmacology, ordinarily second-year programs, the hoped-for increase in basic science learning in the clinical years has not occurred. It has been demonstrated, however, particularly at the School of Basic Medical Sciences in Urbana–Champaign, that one year of carefully planned learning experience is sufficient to prepare most students to pass Part I of the national boards. The school is now developing a clinical curriculum that may provide a greater degree of correlation. Each school has been free to develop its own curriculum, subject to review by and approval of the Academic Council.

Individual School Curricula

The curriculum of the *School of Basic Medical Sciences in Urbana–Champaign* was developed by a team composed of basic scientists who served as content experts, practicing physicians who related curriculum content to clinical problems, and educational specialists who guided the synthesis. Each team defined the elements and skills in a discipline necessary for the practice of scientific medicine, and devised learning experiences in a guided study, problem-oriented mode using clinical problems to complete the coverage of the basic medical sciences. Students are guided in their learning by a syllabus that outlines the educational objectives for each discipline, and computerized self-assessment examinations are available throughout this phase. Patients with specific disease problems are used to demonstrate interdisciplinary principles.

The sequential learning patterns of the traditional medical curriculum have been realigned. Pathology and physical diagnosis, usually covered in the second year of medical school, are introduced in the first week of this program, as the student encounters disease and works from the abnormal to an understanding of the normal. Teaching physical diagnosis at an early stage also takes advantage of the enormous motivation of beginning medical students.

The *School of Basic Medical Sciences at the Medical Center* follows a more traditional curriculum. There is a large degree of interdisciplinary teaching, however, and a syllabus of educational objectives serves as a guide for the students' learning. Unlike the basic sciences school in Urbana–Champaign, objectives were developed by the basic science faculty without consultation with clinicians. Yet a recent survey by faculty members from the two schools revealed an 85 percent overlap in objectives.

The *Abraham Lincoln School of Medicine* is the three-year clinical school at the Medical Center in Chicago. A four-phase curriculum was initiated in 1971: phases I and II cover a period of approximately two academic quarters devoted to the clinical skills of information gathering and problem solving. Special aspects of pathology and pharmacology are reviewed, and such fields as biostatistics, human sexuality, and preventive medicine are among the additional areas of instruction. Phase III, lasting approximately one year, is devoted to traditional eight- to twelve-week clinical clerkships. Phase IV, also a period of approximately one year, is devoted to electives. Students arrange their schedules with the advice of a student-selected advisor. The Abraham Lincoln School of Medicine offers an independent study program in which students, with an advisor, plan their entire curriculum.

The curriculum of the *Rockford School of Medicine* is divided into three phases: 1) basic professional; 2) basic ambulatory; and 3) basic hospital experiences. The professional experience extends over a two-year period and includes educational objectives related to fourteen organ systems. The ambulatory experience is covered in all three years, with the student spending an average of ten half-days a month in small group practices located in rural communities surrounding Rockford. These community health centers provide a learning environment for five second-year, five third-year, and five fourth-year students, each of whom shares responsibility, with an attending physician, for a panel of patients over the three-year period. Basic psychiatry is included in the community health center experience, where student performance may be monitored directly by consulting psychiatrists, or indirectly by videotape with subsequent review by a psychiatrist. The hospital experience occurs during the fourth year and is of approximately eleven months' duration.

The first-year curriculum of the *Peoria School of Medicine* provides an introduction to clinical medicine, emphasizing the patient's social, psychological, and environmental aspects of health. Patient contact allows the student to utilize and expand basic skills in problem solving and to gain insight into the doctor-patient relationship. The second year provides the setting in which supervision of students by primary care physicians places maximum emphasis on the clinical practice of medicine. Learning experiences are provided on the wards of affiliated community hospitals; in family-practice-oriented outpatient units; in offices of physicians in solo practice; in group practice settings; and in a variety of other health agencies and facilities in the community and region. The last year is spent in elective programs.

MAINTENANCE OF QUALITY OF UNDERGRADUATE EDUCATION

As demanded by the original expansion proposal, any plan to increase the output of physicians or modify the curriculum should not compromise the quality of physician graduates. Yet how does one ascertain changes in quality when the parameters used are based on assumptions that have never been tested? The problem facing a faculty attempting to judge the quality of its graduates is almost overwhelming, because there are as yet no generally accepted criteria by which to judge a "good" physician. Although studies have shown little or no correlation between medical school performance and performance in practice, every faculty is called on by its peers to demonstrate "quality." Often the quality of the program is measured in terms of faculty achievements, such as the size of the research budget, number of publications, and membership on prestigious boards and societies, rather than in terms of what the student may have achieved. While these kinds of data may help to describe the environment in which students are supposed to learn, they are not measures of student achievement. Only by establishing educational objectives in advance can sound assessments of student achievement and program quality be made. While all schools of the college have made considerable progress in establishing cognitive objectives, much less has been accomplished in defining non-cognitive goals.

Meanwhile, three commonly used measures of quality are premedical achievement and attitude data, national board examinations results, and attrition rates. Table 1 compares mean grade point averages (GPAs) and Medical College Admission Test (MCAT) scores for the group admitted to the college in 1969 with those of the group admitted in 1974—the last year for which there are complete data. On the achievement criterion, there has been no decrease in the quality of the students admitted. This finding is even

TABLE 1. UNIVERSITY OF ILLINOIS COLLEGE OF MEDICINE:
ADMISSIONS DATA

	September 1969	September 1974
Mean grade point average	4.22	4.47
Medical College Admission Test		
Verbal	561	541
Quantitative	619	615
General information	564	544
Science	589	617

more striking in view of the fact the 11 percent of the 1974 entering class were minority students whose mean GPAs were substantially lower than the remainder of the group. The Committee on Admissions has weighed heavily the MCAT quantitative and science scores in making admissions decisions. Using these parameters, there appears to have been no significant change in the quality of students admitted during the period of curricular transition and the distribution of the students to multiple educational sites.

For twenty-five years all students have been required to take the national board examinations, Parts I and II. Figures 5 and 6 depict the failure rate of Illinois students on these examinations compared with the total United States candidate group over the period 1962–75. While there has been some increase in failures on Part I since 1972, it is no greater than the failure rate in the early 1960s when the curriculum of the college was very stable. Since 1969 an increasing number of minority students have been admitted; the failure rate of this group on national boards, Part I, is higher than that of the remainder of the group. The data presented include all students, but the failure rate on national boards, Part II, varies only slightly from the national average.

No students have been graduated who have not passed both parts of the national boards and the internal comprehensive examinations; they must also have satisfactorily completed all clerkship assignments, where attempts at assessment of noncognitive attributes are made.

The attrition rate from all causes is shown in Figure 7. Attrition, as used here, means students who have left the program for whatever reason and who will never be granted an M.D. degree by the college. The trend is downward, following the national pattern over the past few years.

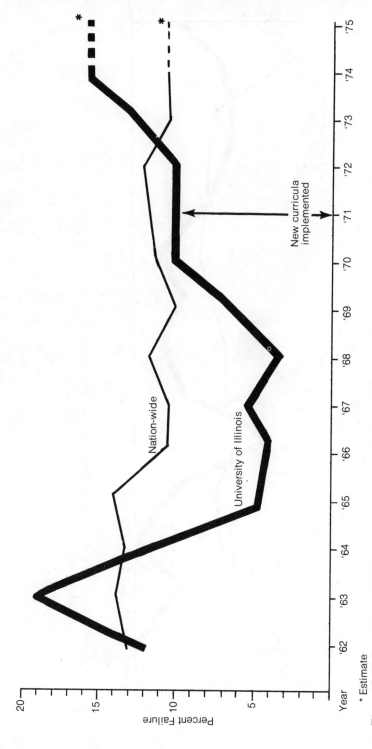

* Estimate

Figure 5. University of Illinois College of Medicine, National Board Results, Part I: Failure Rate of the Candidate Group.

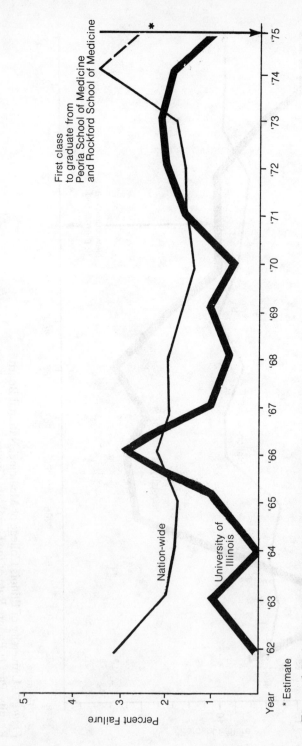

Figure 6. University of Illinois College of Medicine, National Board
Results, Part II: Failure Rate of the Candidate Group.

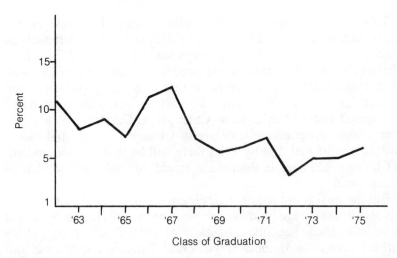

Figure 7. University of Illinois College of Medicine, Attrition Rate, 1962–75.

The current attrition rate for minority group students is about 11.5 percent—somewhat higher than for others. Since such students were not admitted in substantial numbers until 1969, however, it is too early to ascertain a true attrition rate for that group.

MEETING THE OBJECTIVES

It is too soon to assess whether the University of Illinois program is attaining the more detailed objectives it set out to fulfill. Yet in a broad sense the objectives outlined by the faculty in 1968 have been or will be met before too long. At least four hundred M.D. degree candidates will be admitted by 1977, one year beyond the 1976 target date. A system of qualifying examinations has been established that permits normal attrition to be balanced by admission to advanced standing. (Students admitted by this pathway are new entrants to medical school, not transfers from other schools.) The expansion in enrollments has been accommodated through the creation of schools within the college at Peoria, Rockford, Urbana–Champaign, and Chicago. Many new formal affiliation agreements have been negotiated with community hospitals in these areas. Finally, an administrative and faculty organization has been created that allows college faculty to exercise quality control through a system of checks and balances.

Table 2 is a summary of the enrollment data. First-year enrollments increased from 225 in 1969 to 332 in 1975; enrollments in
Chicago, however, rose by only seven students—from 225 to 232.
The additional 100 students are accommodated on the Urbana–
Champaign campus. It is projected that first-year enrollments will
increase to 478 by 1983, with 350 students being accommodated
in Chicago and 128 in Urbana–Champaign. Currently, 928 three-
year clinical program students are in Chicago, Peoria, and Rockford; it is estimated that by 1983 there will be 900 clinical students
in Chicago, 225 each in Peoria and Rockford, and 150 in Urbana–
Champaign.

But the goal is not simply to increase the number of graduates—
it is also to encourage graduates to practice in underserved areas and
to select needed specialties. As early as 1959 Potthoff, in a study
entitled *Trends in Medical Services and Training Facilities in Illinois,* pointed out that physicians tend to practice in the areas where
they take residency training.[12] Prior to 1969 the College of Medicine
sponsored no residency programs outside of the medical center in
Chicago. In 1975 there were thirty family practice residency positions in the Rockford area, twenty in the Peoria area, and five in the
Urbana–Champaign area—a total of fifty-five positions. In addition,
other specialty residency programs are coordinated between the
University Hospital and the Metropolitan Group of Affiliated Hospitals. Figure 8 indicates that the number of students remaining in

TABLE 2. UNIVERSITY OF ILLINOIS COLLEGE OF MEDICINE:
ENROLLMENT DATA

	Actual 1969–70	Actual 1975–76	Projected 1983–84
First year			
Chicago	225	232	350
Urbana–Champaign	0	100	128
Subtotal	(225)	(332)	(478)
Clinical years			
Chicago	595	720	900
Peoria		120	225
Rockford		88	225
Urbana–Champaign		0	150
Subtotal	(595)	(928)	(1,500)
Advanced standing	0	10	22
Total enrollment	820	1,270	2,000

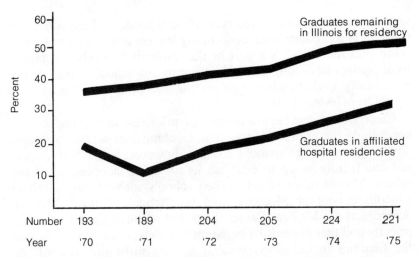

Figure 8. University of Illinois College of Medicine, Residency Selection.

Illinois for residency training rose from 41.6 percent in 1972 to 51.3 percent in 1975.

The three-year family practice residency program at Rockford recently graduated eight physicians, seven of whom stayed on to practice in communities of less than ten thousand population in northwestern Illinois—a bit of evidence that Potthoff's contention may be correct.

PROBLEMS

Problems related to the development of regionalized medical education are similar to those of any expanding school. They fall into four broad categories:

1. Identification with larger institutions—the college, the university, and the local community;

2. Priorities in research, teaching, service, and the associated monetary and academic rewards;

3. Educational philosophy—conflicts of views on curricular organization, instructional methodology, and student evaluation; and

4. Management—the interrelationship of geographically separated campuses with the university bureaucracy, and the relationship of the public to the private sector.

The problem of identification of the new campuses with the college is very real. Sometimes individual schools have sought advantage by soliciting political intervention independent of the college or university; sometimes local community leaders have failed to understand that the school is a part of the university; in other instances local leaders have long delayed accepting the school as part of the community. Perhaps a better public relations program initiated early would have lessened these problems.

Clearly there has been a conflict of priorities among the schools concerning the primacy of research, teaching, and service. A major advantage of the multischool concept, however, is that it does permit one faculty group to establish its priorities independent of the others. The faculties of established schools such as the Abraham Lincoln School of Medicine and the School of Basic Medical Sciences at the Medical Center insist that research should be a first priority and that rewards be based on research productivity, whereas the faculties in the newly created schools insist that rewards be based more on teaching and service. We have tried to deal with the differing priorities realistically through the mechanism of the college level Committee on Faculty Appointments, Promotions, and Tenure. Criteria for promotion and the definition of academic titles are currently being restudied.

The multicampus system permits a variety of educational philosophies to evolve. Each of the schools has different curricular organizations, instructional methods, and content emphasis. Although the instruments of student evaluation for promotional purposes are common to all schools, a continuing issue is the faculty's acceptance of an overall comprehensive examination system. But that problem existed for the first ten years of the system, before the multischool program was implemented, and may relate more to faculty frustration over evaluation of noncognitive qualities than to the examination system per se. The peer review system of each curriculum conducted by the college Committee on Educational Policy is time-consuming, and brings various faculty groups into confrontation over educational issues. The problems thus created are justified, however, in terms of views that are shared, and, one hopes, in terms of the enlightenment of both the traditional faculty and the newer community-based faculty.

Managerial problems relate primarily to the overall size of the University of Illinois and its multiple service units—business office, physical plant, etc.—and to the differences in the modus operandi of public and private institutions. There appears to be no short-term way to prevent interface problems from recurring except through constant renegotiation. Eventually, mutual, enlightened self-interest resolves the issues.

The University of Illinois program strives to create a collegium rather than a loosely bound confederation of schools. The broad problem areas highlighted here have tended to be centrifugal forces pushing the organization toward a confederation. The Administrative Advisory Council, the Academic Council with its subcommittee structure, the centralized budget allocation, the dependence of the clinical schools on the basic science schools, and accreditation requirements are centripetal forces that strengthen the collegial concept.

SUMMARY

Despite many problems, the University of Illinois has within a decade, without extravagant capital expenditure and without sacrifice of student achievement, nearly doubled medical student enrollment; developed multiple schools within the College of Medicine; used existing facilities and staff within the university and the communities as the mechanism for accommodating the increase; created a large minority student program; developed residency programs outside the Chicago metropolitan area; and increased the retention of graduates within the state.

Perhaps most important, three regional centers have been created outside the Chicago metropolitan area that can act as: 1) foci for certain types of graduate education; 2) vehicles for continuing education; and 3) educational components of what I believe to be the emerging regionalized health care delivery system of the United States.

Notes

1. *Physicians for a Growing America,* Report of the Surgeon General's Consultant Group on Medical Education (Washington: U.S. Department of Health, Education, and Welfare, Public Health Service Publication No. 709, 1959).

2. *Health Manpower Source Book* (Washington: U.S. Department of Health, Education, and Welfare, Public Health Service, 1960).

3. Lowell T. Coggeshall, *Planning for Medical Progress Through Education* (Evanston, Illinois: Association of American Medical Colleges, 1965).

4. *The Graduate Education of Physicians,* Report of the Citizens Commission on Graduate Medical Education (Chicago: American Medical Association, 1966).

5. *Meeting the Challenge of Family Practice,* Report of the Ad Hoc Committee on Education for Family Practice of the Council on Medical Education, American Medical Association (Chicago: American Medical Association, 1966).
6. *Health Is a Community Affair,* Report of the National Commission on Community Health Services (Cambridge: Harvard University Press, 1966).
7. "New Directions in Public Policy for Health Care. The 1966 Health Conference," *Bulletin of the New York Academy of Medicine* 42 (December 1966): 1067–1244.
8. E. F. Potthoff, *Trends in Medical Service and Training Facilities in Illinois* (Urbana: University of Illinois Press, 1959).
9. Christine H. McGuire and Lawrence M. Solomon, eds., *Clinical Simulation: Selected Problems in Patient Management* (New York: Appleton Century-Crofts, Educational Division, Meredith Corporation, 1971).
10. James C. Plagge et al., "Increasing the Number of Minority Enrollees and Graduates: A Medical Opportunities Program," *Journal of Medical Education* 49, no. 8 (1974): 735–45.
11. Charles E. Johns and Roger D. Smith, "An Independent Study Program in Medical School," *Journal of Medical Education* 48, no. 8 (1973): 732–38.
12. Potthoff, *Medical Service and Training in Illinois* (see note 8).

DISCUSSION

The discussion opened with a question about the consistency of the community practitioners' commitment to teaching obligations. Grove replied that there had been a sincere desire to avoid a town-gown conflict, and that it had been stipulated at Illinois that any physician could apply for faculty status. There has been a significant attrition rate, but those who remain are deeply committed to teaching. In Rockford and Peoria, for example, while there are no full-time clinical faculty members, many of the community physicians give 50–75 percent of their time to teaching, and they conduct standard clinical clerkships. As to the quality of instruction, the surgical faculty at the main campus believes that the community hospital surgical clerks are as good, if not better, than their peers in Chicago.

To the question of whether the Illinois faculty accepts the necessity for the national boards, Grove answered that at one time there had been serious disagreements on this point, with many feeling that the boards were unnecessary. Today, however, there is an equally strong belief that the school cannot do without the boards. Parts I and II must be taken, and no student who has graduated has failed to pass them.

The National Board of
Medical Examiners

ROBERT A. CHASE *

Since it was established in 1915, the National Board of Medical Examiners (NBME) has been involved in the development of certifying examinations for various segments of the medical profession, and many other types of examinations not designed to certify professional competence. All have been specifically for the medical profession, however, except for one developed in 1972 for the assistant to the primary care physician. This review encompasses three major aspects of the expansion of the NBME: 1) the evolution of policy and function; 2) the growth in services and resources; and 3) current commitments and priority implications.

EVOLUTION OF POLICY AND FUNCTION: 1915–75

With policy issues as a primary focus, the NBME's Policy Advisory Committee found it helpful to view the evolution of policy from the perspective of the changing functions of the NBME over time. Accordingly, policy changes were identified in relation to the functions of examination services, research, and education.

Examination Services

The principal function of the NBME since its creation, and until the 1950s its sole activity, has been the preparation and administration of examinations, so that state medical boards may, at their discretion, accept certified diplomates of the NBME for licensure without further testing. Thus, for the first forty years, the board's

* The material for this survey of the National Board of Medical Examiners was prepared by Edithe J. Levit, M.D., vice-president, NBME, as background information for its Policy Advisory Committee.

responsibility was in the area of undergraduate medical evaluation and licensure.

Over the past two decades the examination services provided by the NBME have been extended along several dimensions (Figure 1). The board first took on the role of a service agency in the early 1950s, when it began to provide its examinations to medical schools for their use in assessing educational achievement. Since these were essentially derived from the regular examinations of the board, this service involved providing a ready-made product, plus the scoring and reporting of results.

Soon thereafter, as organized medicine addressed the confused situation resulting from the influx of foreign medical graduates (FMGs) to the United States, the Educational Council for Foreign Medical Graduates (ECFMG) was established, and the NBME was asked to participate in the design of a screening examination to be given to FMGs who sought internships and residencies in this country. This proposal represented a new departure from the board's traditional function, since it involved the development of a qualifying examination for a purpose other than licensure. After careful deliberation a satisfactory agreement between the two groups was established and the ECFMG gave its first examination in March 1958.

This decision denoted yet another important change with respect to the type of examination services provided, in that, for the first time, the NBME was engaged in creating "custom-made" examinations constructed entirely from its pool of calibrated test questions. A further extension of this service came about with the board's decision in the mid-1960s to collaborate with the Federation of State Medical Boards (FSMB) in developing the Federal Licensing Examination (FLEX), which is also based on test material drawn from the NBME's pool of questions. A similar service has been provided to the Medical Council of Canada (MCC) in the creation of its examinations for licensure. In the latter two instances, while continuing the relationship with licensing boards, the NBME assumed an examination service role quite different from its traditional one as an independent certifying agency.

In 1961 the decision to provide assistance to specialty boards marked the beginning for the NMBE of a new and different service that did not require the use of its own test material. For the first time the board was asked to provide only specific professional and

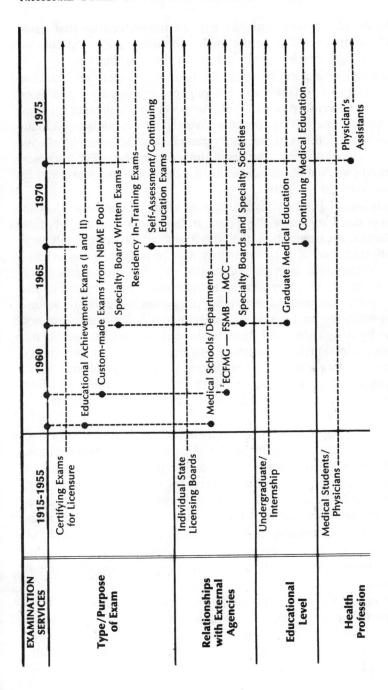

Figure 1. Extension of NBME Examination Services: 1955–75.

administrative services, with the explicit understanding that each specialty board would have the final responsibility for and control over the design, development, and use of the examination.

Providing assistance to specialty boards reflected yet another policy change: the NBME was now engaged in evaluation processes beyond the internship level. Thus, in providing assistance to specialty boards, the NBME became involved in evaluating graduate medical education. As at the undergraduate and licensure levels, its services were soon sought by institutions and agencies for purposes other than certification, for example, the development of in-training examinations for residents.

Beginning in 1967, with the decision of the board to work with the American College of Physicians in the development of its first self-assessment examination, the NBME moved into an entirely new and different area of activity. It was now providing purely educational examination services, unrelated to the measurement of achievement or of individual qualifications. These examinations were to serve the needs of individual physicians, voluntarily assuming responsibility for their own continuing education; they were not utilized by institutions and agencies accountable to the public for assuring professional competence. This activity marked the board's beginning participation in the evaluation process beyond the formal period of undergraduate and graduate medical education, and into the period of continuing education throughout the physician's career.

The foregoing discussion documents the expanding nature and scope of services provided by the NBME over the past two decades. In addition to its own certifying examination, it provides assistance to other certifying and licensing agencies in the development of their own tests. The purposes of these examinations have been extended beyond certification of individual competence, to include educational achievement and in-training examinations, both of which are used as indirect measures of the effectiveness of educational programs, and self-assessment programs for educational purposes.

As a result of these commitments the board's relationships, once confined to individual licensing bodies, now include numerous external agencies and institutions at all levels of medical education: medical schools, the FSMB, the ECFMG, individual specialty boards and societies, as well as other professional organizations and groups. Finally, the board is now engaged in the evaluation process throughout the entire continuum of medical education.

In the course of these rapidly expanding activities, one aspect of the original policy has remained unchanged until recently. From 1915 to 1972 the board's services were provided only to those organizations and agencies concerned with the education, licensure, and certification of physicians. In 1972, based on a strong recommendation from its Goals and Priorities Committee, and following extensive study and consultation, the NBME undertook the responsibility for developing a certifying examination for a new health professional, namely, the assistant to the primary care physician.

While it is beyond the scope of this report to address the many important features of this function, it is important to know that it had the strong endorsement of the American Medical Association (AMA) and its several councils, as well as the endorsement, and indeed the involvement, of several major national medical professional societies. Also, in terms of the board's existing policies, it is of interest to note that the policy adopted in 1967 was included in the following statement of purpose:

> . . . to cooperate with and, where appropriate, to make its specialized services available to the examining boards of the states, specialty boards, and other organizations concerned with the education and qualification of personnel in the fields of health.

Research and Development

While meeting the increasing demands for examination services over the past twenty-five years, the NBME has recognized its responsibility to preserve and extend the quality of its examination procedures, and at the same time to intensify its efforts in developing new and improved testing methods for measuring the knowledge and competence of physicians.

Beginning in the early 1960s with the development of a full-time professional staff with expertise in psychometrics and medicine, the board began to undertake research focused on the improvement of existing examination techniques. Major projects such as the Part III component, the relevance study, and the Computer-Based Examination (CBX) Program were funded through grants from private foundations. At the same time, the board was engaged in a variety of smaller research development efforts related primarily to quality control and validation of existing examination procedures.

Similar studies were carried out in cooperation with various specialty boards for which the NBME was providing examination services. In 1967, based on the recommendation of a special subcommittee of its Executive Committee, the board made a formal commitment to research, as included in the following statement:

> . . . to initiate, develop, and participate in research designed to evaluate the effectiveness of educational programs and techniques, and to assess ever more precisely the knowledge, competence and qualifications of those preparing for and continuing to assume responsibility for the health of the public; . . .

This policy, strongly endorsed by its Goals and Priorities Committee, was formally implemented in 1973 with the establishment of a Department of Research and Development, through which the NBME has embarked on a major research effort related to the assessment of professional competence. The growth in research, as reflected in extramural funding, is shown in Figure 2.

Education

The NBME's educational role has essentially been informal and unstructured. Education in the field of evaluation and measurement has been conducted mainly as a supportive activity to improve the process of test development. To this end the board has provided such educational opportunities through its meetings with various examination committees, as well as through consultation with a number of professional groups and the Annual Invitational Conference. The board's commitment to this activity was recognized in 1967 with the revision of its bylaws to include the following purpose:

> . . . to provide educational opportunities for professional personnel in the methods, techniques and values of testing methods related to knowledge and competence in the broad field of medicine.

To date the board has not implemented this policy in a formal way. New proposals for the development of educational and training programs have, however, recently been made to the Executive Committee by the professional staff.

PATTERNS OF GROWTH IN SERVICES AND RESOURCES: 1950–75

Traditionally, the growth pattern of the NBME has been viewed in terms of the total number of examinations processed each year,

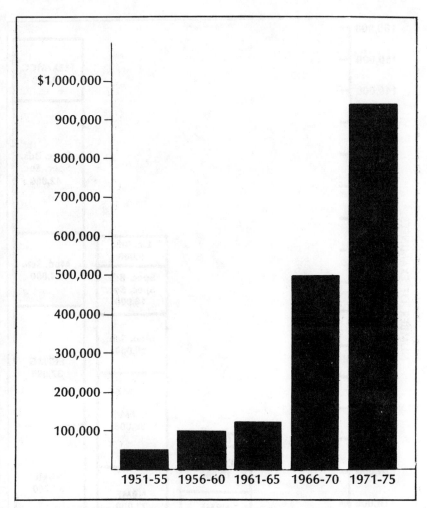

Figure 2. NBME Extramural Research Funds: 1950–75.

which is essentially a reflection of the number of individuals examined. Figure 3 shows the cumulative total, as well as the sub-
total, for the various types of examinations over the past twenty-five
years.

In further consideration of the types of examinations shown in
Figure 3, the growth in certain categories, such as the NBME and
the ECFMG, was based solely on the increasing numbers of individuals examined. The growth in services to specialty boards and

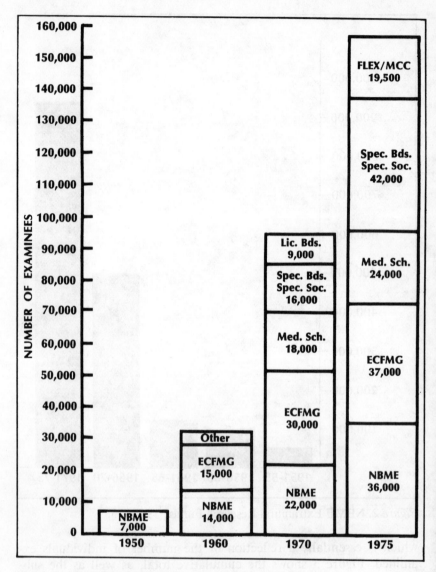

Figure 3. NBME Examination Services: 1950–75.

specialty societies as shown for 1970 and 1974, however, primarily reflected not only an increase in the number of individual boards and societies requesting NBME assistance in the development of their respective examinations, but multiple new programs for some of the agencies. The principal effort required to design and implement a new examination program was essentially independent of the number who might ultimately take the examination: the professional effort is the same whether it is given to one thousand or ten thousand individuals.

CURRENT COMMITMENTS OF THE NBME

Analysis of growth patterns over the past twenty-five years proved the point that the NBME's commitments could not be measured by examining allocations of operating budget, space, and supporting staff to various services. The most reasonable composite of the board's commitments is best derived from the total effort of the professional staff to services. Data was collected by means of the analysis and calculation of composite effort devoted to each category of activity.

Total professional staff effort is illustrated in Figure 4, which shows that 51.8 percent of professional staff time is devoted to examination services; 26.2 percent to research and development; and the remaining 21.9 percent to overall NBME administration and consultant "educational" activities.

As shown in Figure 5, 69.8 percent of the professional staff effort

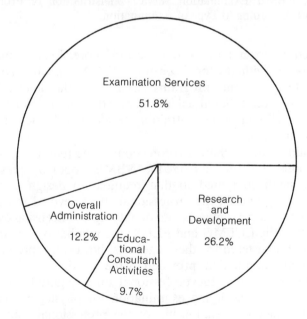

Figure 4. Distribution of Total NBME Professional Staff Effort.

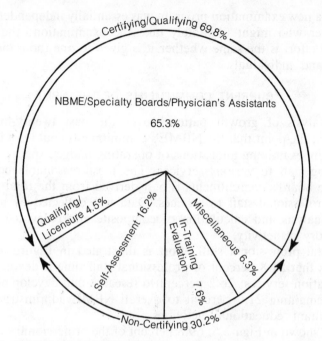

Figure 5. NBME Examination Services: Distribution of Professional Staff Effort According to Type of Examination.

is devoted to examinations that certify professional competence or qualify individuals for licensure (FLEX) or for admission to graduate educational programs (ECFMG); the other 30.2 percent relates to educational achievement, educational programmatic evaluation, self-education, in-training resident evaluation, and miscellaneous activities.

It should be noted that the professional time required to develop examinations constructed from the NBME's pool of questions is relatively small compared to that required to design a new examination program. Of the professional effort devoted to examination services, 4.5 percent goes into qualifying and licensing examinations such as the ECFMG and FLEX; the number of examinations (56,500) administered for these agencies, however, represents 37.1 percent of all examinations provided by the board.

On the other hand, the professional time required for the development of the certifying examination for physician's assistants (PAs) illustrates the relationship of the professional staff and its activities to a new program. Comparable data are not available for the initial year of this program. For the second year, however, it is estimated that 8 percent of professional staff time devoted to examination services went into the PA examination. While professional staff effort is nearly double that required for the FLEX and the ECFMG, the number of examinations administered in the PA program (1,300) represents only 0.9 percent of the total provided by the board.

Professional Staff Time Devoted to Certifying Examinations

It is of interest to note that of professional staff time devoted to certifying examinations, the largest commitment is to the specialty boards in the area of graduate medical education (Figure 6). At present the NBME assists twelve of the twenty-two primary boards in the design of written certifying examinations for the specialty boards. Also, of the sixteen subspecialty boards that require an oral examination as part of the certification process, the NBME is currently helping three of them in the development and analysis of such examinations.

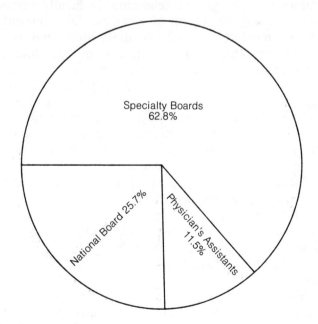

Figure 6. NBME Staff Time Devoted to Certifying Examinations.

With the advent of recertification assessment procedures, the relationship of the NBME with the specialty boards will inevitably expand. The board is now consulting with one specialty board in creating a recertification examination. At the same time it is assisting six specialty societies in the preparation of self-assessment programs, an activity that may very well ultimately relate to the recertification process.

The progressive increase in the NBME's involvement with specialty boards and societies since 1961, together with the other activities already noted, suggests that the board can anticipate additional requests for its examination and research services in the future.

THE NBME'S RELATIONSHIP TO
SCHOOLS OF MEDICINE

The core activity of the NBME since it was founded has depended on its relationship to schools of medicine in the United States and Canada.

The focus and content of the board's own Parts I, II, and III examinations have always been determined by faculty members representing essentially all schools of medicine. Development of test materials and regular review of previously used items are carried out by faculty-constituted test committees from other disciplines.

Medical students help determine the performance characteristics of test items on the examinations. The psychometric analysis to determine reliability and question difficulty, for example, depends on overall student performance on the items, and performance by specific reference groups of students. The end result is a fully calibrated test item for predictable use in designing and constructing future examinations for various purposes.

The NBME thus relies on medical school faculty and students for the health of its examinations. The schools of medicine rely on the expertise of the NBME professional and support staff to help assure test validity and reliability; to consult on the use of new evaluation methodology; to carry out professional scoring and analysis; and to guarantee production and administration of top quality examinations.

This interdependence offers the schools the opportunity to use appropriate externally devised evaluation materials, generated by a broad representative group of faculty members from a large number of medical schools, and refined by evaluation professionals, to measure the educational achievements of their students, as compared with others. Such a relationship offers a student an index of his own performance on a comparative basis. This has become more important for the student who intends to practice medicine, and an additional responsibility for faculty test committee members, since NBME test material is now used as a measure of one qualification for licensure by essentially all states. Medical licensure currently requires, among other things, a passing score on board examinations and certification, or on the FLEX, which is constituted entirely of calibrated NBME test items. The responsibility lies, as it should, with medical educators in the United States in partnership with high-quality, professional assessment experts.

Use of NBME tests by students and schools of medicine has been incremental in the last two decades. Students may elect to sit for board examinations for comparative assessment or as one route to practice licensure. The schools have variously used the examinations as external measures of their students' educational progress. Some schools (79 percent in 1974) require students to take Part I, Part II, or both, but do not demand a passing grade standard; in others, students have to take and pass the examination at the NBME standard—Part I, 17 percent of the schools; Part II, 29 percent; in still others, students do not need to take the examinations.

Whether or not students take the examinations, it is clear that approximately 87 percent of them sit for Part I; 84 percent for Part II; and 79 percent for Part III, leading to licensure. (The data cannot be absolutely precise because students from various classes take Parts I and II, and because those taking Part III in any given year do not all graduate from medical school at the same time.) Even those students who do not take the board examinations, do take the FLEX in order to become licensed. Thus essentially all individuals who practice medicine in the United States must take an examination, the content of which is in part determined by medical school faculty.

Medical school faculty members have been asking with increasing frequency for subject tests from the NBME. The prospect is that in the years ahead the NBME will be able to make the test material more accessible for such tailor-made examinations, using nationally calibrated test items designed to measure the achievement of students in a given course of study. The computerized test-item library system, now close to the implementation level, will be of inestimable value for individual faculty development of specially tailored tests.

It is and will continue to be the intention of the NBME to reflect changes in knowledge and in curriculum while maintaining a national standard, as viewed by a composite of medical faculty; it is not the board's intention to determine curriculum specifically, as long as students by some means gain the minimum measurable competence required for acquisition of the certificate.

Medical schools are free to use the standard board examinations as they see fit, with limitations on security and confidentiality. In the future the combined medical schools' test materials at NBME will be more accessible for individualized examination construction.

NBME RESEARCH AND DEVELOPMENT EFFORTS

The current emphasis in research and development at the NBME is on methodology to measure reliably the noncognitive competencies that clearly are component essentials for the proper practice of medicine. Emphasis on performance, as well as on knowledge, is evident in the techniques under study. A sample of some of the studies currently underway demonstrate areas under exploration.

1. The Interpersonal Skills Project is designed to measure and predict physician behavior in interactions with patients, colleagues, and others. This attempt to prove whether or not such skills are subject to objective measure uses direct and indirect methodology: a) the skills are being defined, and an attempt is being made to show a relationship between skills and outcome; b) use of professionally designed rating scales, and interactions between candidates and actors are under study; c) candidate responses to videotaped patient-physician interactions constitute an indirect approach; d) written protocols depicting clinical situations and interactions, combined with responses to multiple-choice questions are being tested.

2. Audiovisual simulations, as a step closer to practice reality and a measurement of candidate response, are at the prototype stage as another means of measuring performance.

3. Assessment of physical examination skills, already tested and found reliable in the examination, has implications for the evaluation of many important combined intellectual and motor skills.

4. Medical audit projects to evaluate performance are underway.

Obviously audit systems are only as good as the medical records generated, as Lawrence Weed has pointed out. Nonetheless, the record is a look at process performance, and a partial display of outcome for the individual patients related to the physician candidate's performance.

5. Computer-Based Examination (CBX) research will likely provide new and practical measures of physician competence. Just as the computer is gaining importance as an instrument useful in education, so is it becoming a useful new tool in evaluation. A major project is jointly being carried out, sponsored by the NBME and the American Board of Internal Medicine, to develop CBX to an operational level.

6. Rating scale projects, physician profile studies strategic to enhance oral examinations, and motor skill evaluations are among other methodologies currently under study by NBME staff, in some cases with other organizations.

Some of these methodologies are particularly appropriate to a major project of the NBME—the development of a comprehensive qualifying examination appropriate for use in the transition from undergraduate to graduate education. The purpose is to assure that candidates entering graduate medical education have those measurable components of competence considered essential to one assuming responsibility for patient care in a graduate setting.

FUTURE USE OF NBME RESOURCES

In response to a growing number of requests for the NBME's services from a variety of organizations, at the request of the Board of Directors the board chairman appointed a Policy Advisory Committee. The committee's deliberations and recommendations were recently presented to the NBME Executive Committee. They displayed a well-thought-through set of priorities that considered the implications of implementing priority guidelines. Although a first priority of the NBME under the guidelines would continue to be a commitment of resources to recognized agencies and institutions responsible for *education, licensure,* and *certification* of physicians, the guidelines would permit a reasonable extension of services to allied health groups whose educational programs are accredited by the proposed Joint Council on Accreditation of Allied Health Education or a similar body.

The Policy Advisory Committee supported and urged development of combined NBME–university educational programs for professionals interested in advancing their qualifications to participate in evaluation of competence in medicine. Other exciting proposals for future initiatives by NBME were also suggested.

It is the objective of the NBME to serve where its unique resources are required, and to maintain a high quality of performance so that standards in medicine may reliably be set in the best interests of both the profession and the public.

DISCUSSION

Weed outlined of what he considered to be the task of the National Board of Medical Examiners. Among the points he made were:

- Medical schools would state what they expect from their students in the way of proper patient care; this would include a problem list, statement of plans, etc.
- The schools would clarify the respective roles in the hierarchy of students, house staff, and faculty in the examination process.
- Examiners would visit the schools at random with a list of those students who wished to obtain credentials. The examiners would study the records of patients for whom the students were responsible and assess them for their thoroughness, reliability, and analytical soundness. If a half-dozen of a student's records were satisfactory, he would receive his credentials.
- In a similar fashion, practicing physicians would be checked at random throughout their careers.

A number of participants, while admiring the intent of Weed's proposals, felt that it was not possible to implement them in the "real world." Weed replied that, instead, it would be better to ask what the "real world" needs and use our ingenuity to produce it.

Turning to the national boards, some discussants agreed that the proper emphasis had in fact been placed on the board examinations as tools of those who use them. To use the tests properly, the faculty must define what they expect of them. They may, for example, be useful as red flags: if 30 percent of the first-year students fail the pharmacology section of Part I, the faculty will be alerted that there is a deficiency in pharmacology instruction. On balance, testing should play the least important part in student evaluation, and tutorial assessment the largest role.

The national boards are supposed to be norm-based, but in effect they are criterion-based, because the reference group for Part I is composed of selected first-time takers who have completed the first two years of medical school. They form a relatively pure group from which, using their scores, a curve is determined. A cutting score, based on this curve, is then established for the balance of the examinations.

There is a feeling that the boards should be criterion-based, but this is not easy to accomplish. For example, the obstetrics-gynecology test committee attempted to introduce such an examination. The committee criterion-referenced the test by selecting several questions that had to be answered. A number of students who had, in general, performed in a superior manner, missed one or two of the questions, however, and thus failed the entire examination.

The overall issue of the role of the national boards and the Princeton testing group is vitally important for medical education and education is general. Several participants argued that this issue, along with that of the high cost of medical care, are the two most important problems in medicine today.

A number of the discussants expressed the opinion that the multiple-choice test, given repeatedly, is not really an objective examination but a rite of passage that students will pass if they know they must. The National Board of Medical Examiners can predict the mean score on its examination quite easily: with twenty thousand questions in its computer, it can change the ratio of the hardest questions, making the test easier or more difficult, and thus raising or lowering the mean score. Some see this as the "tyranny" of the national boards. Others, while conceding that weaknesses do exist, felt it is better not to scrap the entire system when no viable alternatives have been suggested.

Problems in Evaluation
and Examination

JOHN C. HERWEG

Initially I viewed by assignment to speak on "Problems in Evaluation and Examination" as an aggressive act by some unknown colleague. With the passage of time, reflective thought, and some degree of resignation, however, I decided this assignment would give me an opportunity to voice my views and opinions on the subject. Indeed it seemed attractive to have thirty, consecutive, uninterrupted minutes to expound on this topic, since in more than ten years' service as an ex officio member on my school's Committee on Medical Education I have never enjoyed such a privilege.

At the outset, I claim no special expertise in the fields of psychological testing, human behavorial analysis, educational psychology, or computers. I hasten to state, however, that based on over thirty years experience as a medical student, intern, military physician, resident physician, pediatric practitioner, medical school faculty member, would-be researcher, and administrator I have developed strong opinions, and probably much bias, on these subjects, and I welcome the opportunity to share them with you.

The current climate for evaluation and examination is favorable. This is true at all levels: public, private, local, national, and international. Many events and circumstances—the long, agonizing Vietnamese conflict; the Watergate affair; the concern about our environment; the energy crisis; the inexorable rise in crime; the changing mores; the civil rights and women's liberation movements; the approaching bicentennial—all of these and more have stimulated us, if not forced us, to reflect, review, dissect, rethink, regret, and finally to plan and resolve to commit ourselves and our energies to new directions and new goals. This mood was well stated by David Matthews, the new secretary of the Department of Health, Education, and Welfare, when he described the last decade as "the age when things didn't work out like we thought they would," adding that "the great obligation in such a time is to reassessment and reevaluation and to a common rethinking." [1]

In the broad field of medicine this type of analysis and rethinking has occurred and is continuing to occur in multiple areas: in the premedical educational sphere; in the selection process for admission of students; in the content and sequence of undergraduate medical education; in postgraduate residency and fellowship training; in medical licensure; in medical records; in specialty certification; and in the maintenance of professional competency. A brief glimpse at each of these areas should provide us with a background and perspective with which we can view some of the current problems in evaluation and examination.

PREMEDICAL EDUCATION

In the immediate post-*Sputnik* period a major national goal was to beat the Russians to the moon. Great emphasis was placed on science, engineering, and technology, with the result that our nation's secondary schools, colleges, and universities took a hard look at their science curricula. This was rapidly followed by a marked upgrading in the quality of course content and in the diversity of courses available in biology, chemistry, physics, and engineering. Many bright young men and women were attracted to these fields, and science literally blossomed.

This receptive environment and the encouraging financial support from governmental and private sources resulted in an information explosion, particularly in biology and the biomedical sciences. As a consequence, the scientific background of many of today's entering medical students is extremely sophisticated. There is still, however, considerable heterogeneity as regards their exposure to and competence in the sciences basic to medicine.

MEDICAL SCHOOL ADMISSIONS

Undergraduate schools, medical schools, and applicants are today spending tremendous amounts of time, effort, and money in the process of selecting this nation's future physicians. The material and human wastage that occurs in a process whereby only one out of three applicants is successful requires, if not demands, better systems of both undergraduate school career counseling and medical school applicant evaluation.

The Medical College Admission Test (MCAT) was initially designed to facilitate the selection of students who would succeed in passing the basic science coursework in the medical school curriculum. Concurrent with, but not necessarily as a result of, its use, medical school attrition has dropped progressively from an unacceptable 15 percent [2] to its present low level of 1.4 percent.

The Medical College Admissions Assessment Program (MCAAP) is a promising outgrowth of the MCAT program, prompted by the generally-agreed-upon need for a more effective, reliable, and informative test instrument, with superior predictability, to assist in the selection of students. Strong support for the MCAAP from the Group on Student Affairs, the Group on Medical Education, the Organization of Student Representatives, and the Council of Deans of the Association of American Medical Colleges (AAMC), the Association of Advisors for the Health Professions, and other interested bodies has provided grass-roots input. The test program, which is expected to be available in the spring of 1977, focuses on cognitive areas, and should provide information about the applicant's abilities in reading comprehension, problem solving, and specific skills in the fields of biology, chemistry, physics, and mathematics. Following the implementation of this phase of the MCAAP, the many-fold, more difficult problem of developing and validating test instruments to assess noncognitive aspects of medical school applicants will I hope, be addressed promptly and aggressively.

UNDERGRADUATE MEDICAL EDUCATION

Twenty-five to thirty years ago the curricula of the nation's medical schools were very similar if not identical. Curricular revisions initiated in the early 1950s at the Western Reserve University School of Medicine were followed by major changes in essentially every medical school in the United States. Many new schools, uninhibited by restricting tradition, developed innovative curricula based on the premise that learning consisted of behavioral modification, and that educational goals and objectives could be developed and tests devised to determine whether or not students had achieved the stated objectives.

Curricular changes in most medical schools have permitted earlier clinical contact for students; increased elective opportunities; encouraged earlier choice of career direction; allowed individualized curricula; and utilized teaching devices such as programmed texts, audiovisual aids, and computer-assisted learning in addition to the familiar lecture-seminar format.

POSTGRADUATE EDUCATION

Evaluation of postgraduate and fellowship training programs has resulted in the elimination of free-standing internships and better coordination of undergraduate and graduate medical education as a continuum. Some effort, but not enough, has been made in the direction of structuring residency training programs to prepare many young physicians for effective practice, and a much smaller number for careers in academic medicine or administration. Most residency programs continue to emphasize the care of the seriously ill, hospitalized patient, providing little experience in the care of outpatients or instruction in the types of clinical problems residents will encounter in practice.

Care of patients served by many of our university medical centers remains fragmented and lacks longitudinal continuity. There is obvious need for continued examination and evaluation of postgraduate medical training if medicine is to fulfill society's needs and expectations.

MEDICAL LICENSURE

The issue of medical licensure has recently been undergoing close scrutiny from within and outside the medical profession. Medical licensure, which traditionally has been a state's right, is moving toward increasing uniformity of testing procedures and, it is hoped, evaluation of competence. The Goals and Priorities Report of the National Board of Medical Examiners (NBME)[3] reflects the type of self-examination and assessment by concerned members of the profession that one hopes will deter federal imposition of restrictive licensing regulations, which most probably would be administered by nonprofessional bureaucrats.

MEDICAL RECORDS

The Problem-Oriented Medical Record (POMR), which emphasizes the logical and efficient collection of medical data on each patient,[4] has been developed at a time when physicians and hospitals are essentially being forced by the government and by third-party payers to evaluate and control more effectively both the quality and cost of medical care. The POMR system provides for the organized collection of data; the listing of a patient's problem or problems; the formulation of diagnostic plans and treatment appropriate for each problem; and detailed follow up of each of the designated problems by descriptive progress notes. The system leads to a greater uniformity and completeness of medical records; provides for a more efficient means of communication between members of the health care team; and facilitates computerization of information.

Professional Standards Review Organizations (PSROs). Throughout the nation, PSROs, as required by recent federal legislation (Public Law 92–603), are in various stages of development. The PSRO regulations are similar in scope to federal laws that already govern utilization review and medical audit for patients receiving Medicare and Medicaid benefits. The concerted and conscientious efforts of hospital staff members and administrators across the country will be necessary to make this system work. It may well be the one and only opportunity the medical profession has to continue to maintain control over patient care. Upgrading the quality of medical care and providing high-quality service uniformly to all, in the context of cost control, are mandatory essentials at a time when this country is rapidly approaching a system of federally subsidized health care for all citizens.

SPECIALTY RECERTIFICATION

The more than twenty medical specialty boards have played a significant role in improving the quality of education in the specialties and in providing excellent medical care in their respective fields. Physician certification by these boards has in the past conferred "specialist status" on the physician throughout his or her professional career.

In recent years some specialty boards have developed voluntary self-assessment programs for their members. It is reasonable to expect that these will evolve into required reassessment programs, which, together with mandatory attendance at postgraduate courses and, perhaps, practice audit, will constitute the essentials of a periodic specialty recertification procedure.

RELICENSURE

At present, medical licensure is awarded by the various states to those physicians who successfully pass the necessary examinations and other requirements as established by the legally constituted boards of the healing arts. Short of committing a felony or a similar serious unprofessional act, a physician once licensed is so privileged for the rest of his professional career merely upon payment of a small annual fee. It seems reasonable to anticipate that in the future, analogous to what probably will occur in specialty recertification, periodic demonstration of professional competence will be a requisite for continuing medical licensure.

* * * *

All of these briefly mentioned topics may now serve as a backdrop for a discussion of some of the problems in evaluation and examination we were asked to address. And indeed there *are* problems, most of which are difficult of solution, and some probably unsolvable.

Initially, as with many problems, there is the matter of *inertia*. Why should medical schools change their approach to teaching and evaluating medical students when their present methods produce such fine end products? American medicine is the best in the world —or at least we would like to think so. Medical students are, for the most part, extremely competent young men and women, as indeed they ought to be, having been selected from such a large qualified applicant pool. They are mature, strongly motivated, and very resilient. Most of them feel a strong sense of responsibility for their own education. Medical students will learn even in a less-than-optimum learning environment. As long as the system works reasonably well there will be some, and usually many, faculty members in each medical school who are reluctant to alter the status quo. Inertia is indeed a problem.

A medical school has many responsibilities other than strictly educational ones. The complexities and demands of patient care, the vicissitudes of research and its funding, the frustrations of administering a university hospital and of dealing with the multiple problems of the faculty consume most of the time and effort of the dean and department heads. Even though the dean fills a leadership role in medical education, the short duration in office of the average dean may preclude continuity of interest and support. At the other extreme, the long tenure of some departmental chairpersons may tend to inhibit and block curricular changes.

At least some, and probably many, medical schools lack educational leadership. It is very easy to decide, "Let's do what we did last year." When educational responsibility is delegated to interested young faculty members, progress is often limited and compromised without strong support of the power structure. Medical schools with strong departmental organization and autonomy often are unable or unwilling to coordinate their educational and evaluative programs into a logical and meaningful continuum for students. This may result in unnecessary duplication and redundancy; important areas of omission; inconsistent standards of performance; and uncertainty as to whether or not students are meeting these standards.

Most medical school faculty members have had no formal training in the area of education. They are unaware of or unwilling to accept the fact that there is a body of knowledge concerning how people learn and how to assist and monitor that learning. Faculty members are usually recruited and hired because of their research and/or clinical expertise, not for their competence in teaching and medical education. Some are inherently great teachers; a few are disasters, and should not be given educational responsibilities. The majority of new medical school faculty members develop teaching expertise and evaluative competence gradually, largely by trial and error. A short, annual, concisely presented course in educational techniques, educational philosophy, and evaluative methodology, with required attendance by all new faculty members, might well accelerate their adjustment as productive and skilled educators.

The system of rewards in the majority of medical schools is based on research productivity, as indicated by the number of research papers published; grantsmanship, as reflected by the dollar value of grants received; and clinical expertise, as shown by the ledger total of clinical practice income. It is much more difficult to quantitate the quality and success of teaching, and the sincerity and depth of the physician-patient relationship. Although one sees gradual positive changes in the rewards system, it is still probably unwise for a young, untenured faculty member to spend too much time in teaching pursuits if he is looking primarily for rapid academic career development and advancement.

EXPENDITURES FOR RESEARCH AND
DEVELOPMENT IN MEDICAL EDUCATION

The determination of the cost of educating an undergraduate medical student in any of our medical teaching centers is difficult, if not impossible. In the clinical training period, especially, the separation of the cost of education from that of research and patient service is obviously a very arbitrary one. On the basis of two recent educational cost studies,[5, 6] if one accepts the figure of $12,500 as a reasonable annual per capita cost estimate, and if there were approximately fifty-three thousand five hundred medical students in the United States in 1974–75, then the annual undergraduate medical educational bill amounts to a staggering $669 million. If medical education is a business, and it seems to be a big business, it would appear reasonable to invest money in educational research and development with the hope of improving efficiency and reducing costs. In a profit-motivated business, a minimum of 5 percent of profits, and sometimes much more, is invested annually in research and development. Should not comparable amounts be invested by nonprofit-making educational institutions?

In the 1974–75 academic year, forty of our schools of medicine had no unit responsible for research in and development of the education process. In the remaining seventy-four schools this responsibility was delegated to a variety of individuals, units, and groups, ranging from an assistant dean for curriculum, to curriculum committees of faculty and students, to full departments or divisions of research in medical education. There is obviously a wide spectrum of energy, money, and professional talent expended in this area in the medical schools.

EDUCATIONAL GOALS AND OBJECTIVES

In the education of a future physician, lawyer, engineer, minister, teacher, or whatever, it seems fundamental that those responsible for the teaching program set certain goals and objectives to be attained at each stage of the educational process. These may be both short term, such as might be developed for an undergraduate medical school course, and long term, based on performance criteria of the end product, in this case a practicing physician. It follows automatically that only after goals and objectives have been established can a valid system of examination and evaluation be developed.

In 1974 some statement of behavioral-learning objectives was required in sixty-eight of the nation's medical schools, but only twenty-nine published these statements. Such reports were not required in the remaining forty-six schools.[7] I suppose educational goals and objectives have not been established for a host of reasons: 1) it is not easy to do; 2) it requires considerable faculty interest, time, and effort; 3) it requires faculty cooperation and educational leadership; 4) it requires diligent implementation; and 5) it demands frequent review and revision. Nevertheless, I contend that reasonable goals and objectives for medical education must be established by the profession—otherwise they will be established for us.

EDUCATIONAL MEASURING DEVICES

Without doubt the major obstacle standing in the path of progress in evaluation and examination in all aspects of medicine is the lack of appropriate, validated measuring devices. Medical educators, psychologists, behavioral scientists, academic physicians, medical practitioners, resident physicians, medical students, premedical students, college professors, and the consumers of health care—the general public—all have important contributions to make to this complex problem or series of problems. Despite the efforts of many, however, some of the problems of evaluation may be unsolvable. What may seem to be appropriate and reasonable evaluative measures for one group in one locale at one time, may be partially or entirely inappropriate and fallacious for another group in another locale, even at the same time. It would seem logical, in Mattson's words, that: "Examining a person's knowledge, skills and judgment in relation to a task which he will be required to perform seems to be the only sensible way to attack the problem of assessing competence." He hastens to add, however, that ". . . criterion-related measures in education are almost universally a delusion, and that, in fact, virtually all assessment in education can be found under close scrutiny, to be based on performance related to the performance of a norming group."[8] Obviously much work, innovative and imaginative in nature, and both short-term and long-term in scope, must be focused on this complex and challenging problem area. The public, and especially federal and state legislators, must not be led to believe that evaluation and assessment of competence can be solved in a simplistic fashion.

*   *   *   *

So far we have listed some of the issues in the area of evaluation and examination. To list and even to classify problems is merely an exercise in frustration, unless, by looking at them, solutions, or at least attempts at solutions, are forthcoming. So how do we solve these problems? I would suggest the following:

1. Medical schools and teaching hospitals need to place increasing emphasis on the educational aspects of their programs.

2. Leadership in medical education must be provided by the power structure of these institutions. The appropriate investment of time by faculty, education specialists, and students is essential to progress in the evaluation of competency. Such investment must be rewarded above and beyond the mere self-gratification of the participants.

3. Institutions, foundations, and governments must provide the necessary funding for well-devised, evaluative experiments in medical education.

4. Despite the fact that some decry criterion-related measurements, it seems only appropriate to educate and evaluate medical professionals to perform in a competent and compassionate fashion the multitude of tasks they will encounter in their three- to four-decade careers.

5. Time is of the essence. The control of the medical profession is passing almost inexorably from professionals to those who, increasingly, are paying the cost—namely the government and third-party payers. Medicine must play a strong and aggressive leadership role in the education, evaluation, and geographic and specialty distribution of health professionals, so that high-quality health care is accessible and available to all members of society.

The gauntlet is thrown; the stakes are almost incomprehensible; the opportunities are mind-boggling. Medicine must accept the challenge, and by our individual and collective performances we must justify continuing public trust.

Notes

1. D. Matthews, Speech at swearing-in ceremony as Secretary of Health, Education, and Welfare, Washington, D.C., 8 August 1975.
2. D. G. Johnson and E. B. Hutchins, "Doctor or Dropout?: A Study of Medical Student Attrition," *Journal of Medical Education* 41, no. 9 (1966): 1099–1269.
3. National Board of Medical Examiners, *Evaluation in the Continuum of Medical Education,* Report of the Committee on Goals and Priorities of the

National Board of Medical Examiners (Philadelphia: National Board of Medical Examiners, 1973).

4. L. L. Weed, *Medical Records, Medical Education and Patient Care* (Cleveland, Ohio: Case Western Reserve University Press, 1969).

5. *Cost of Education in the Health Professions* (Washington: Institute of Medicine, National Academy of Sciences, 1974).

6. "Undergraduate Medical Education: Elements, Objectives, Costs," Report of the Committee on the Financing of Medical Education of the American Medical Association, *Journal of Medical Education,* 49, no. 1, suppl. (1974): 97–128.

7. *1974–75 Association of American Medical Colleges Curriculum Directory* (Washington: Association of American Medical Colleges, 1975).

8. D. E. Mattson, "Criterion-Related Measures in Education," *Journal of Medical Education* 46, no. 3 (1971): 185–89.

Developments in Graduate
Medical Education

WILLIAM D. HOLDEN

Graduate medical education in the United States is undergoing change as a result of the acceptance of two basic principles that have been addressed only casually in the past. First is a developing realization that graduate education in medicine cannot remain a distinct and separate entity from undergraduate and continuing education, with multiple autonomous and frequently competing organizations and individuals sharing the responsibility and authority for education, accreditation, and certification. Second is an increasing awareness that all categories of medical education are a prelude to the provision of health care and that educational objectives, content, and patterns must adapt to the real or even alleged needs of society.

The following is a brief discussion of some of the principal and interrelated changes occurring in graduate medical education.

FAMILY PRACTICE

In the mid-1950s the Council on Medical Education (CME) of the American Medical Association (AMA) became concerned about the decreasing number of general practitioners and their lack of any well-defined graduate education. Following a study in conjunction with the Association of American Medical Colleges (AAMC) and the American Academy of General Practice, two-year residencies in general practice were established with the approval of the CME.

By 1964 there were seventeen residency programs approved in hospitals affiliated with schools of medicine, and 141 in unaffiliated hospitals.[1] A total of 767 residency positions were offered. Three hundred and seventy-seven were filled, of which 237, or 63 percent were occupied by foreign medical graduates, and 140, or 37 percent,

253

by graduates of American schools. In the same year there were 73,144 general practitioners—26 percent of the physicians in the United States.

By 1973 the number of residency programs in general practice approved by the AMA had dwindled from 258 to fifty-one, seventeen of them in affiliated hospitals. Of the 343 residency positions, 250 were filled, fifty-three of them, or 21 percent, by American graduates. The number of general practitioners had fallen to 53,946, or 14.7 percent of the total physician population.[2] One of the significant factors contributing to the failure of general practice residencies was the absence of board certification.

The obvious lack of interest in these residencies on the part of graduating medical students became apparent by 1964, at which time the CME appointed the Committee on Education in Family Practice. Its report in 1966 defined family practice as a new specialty with characteristics quite distinct from existing concepts of general practice. The report defined the family physician as

> . . . one who 1) serves as the physician of first contact with the patient and provides a means of entry into the health care system; 2) evaluates the patient's total health needs, provides personal medical care within one or more fields of medicine, and refers the patient when indicated to appropriate sources of care while preserving the continuity of his care; 3) assumes responsibility for the patient's comprehensive and continuous health services; and 4) accepts responsibility for the patient's total health care within the context of his environment, including the community and the family or comparable social unit.[3]

The report recommended that a specialty board be established to certify family practitioners after completion of a three-year residency. Residency programs were established in the late 1960s, and in 1969 the American Board of Family Practice (ABFM) was established.

By July 1975, 232 residency programs in family practice had been approved by the Residency Review Committee in Family Practice and the Liaison Committee on Graduate Medical Education. These programs provided approximately sixteen hundred first-year positions. By 1975, 7,073 physicians had been certified by the ABFM. Many of these were general practitioners who qualified to take the certifying examinations; progressively, more are graduates of approved residencies in family practice.

The rapid growth of this specialty appears to be the result of a recognition by graduating students of the concept of a family practitioner as a personal physician to his patients, in contrast to the organ- and systems-oriented practice characteristic of most specialists.

In developing residency programs in family practice many problems have arisen, especially in university medical centers. Departments of medicine and, to a lesser extent, department of pediatrics have expressed concern that the family practitioner will displace the general internist and general pediatrician. As a result, the expansion of residencies in family practice in university hospitals and the establishment of departments of family medicine in medical schools have proceeded slowly. By 1975, however, eighty-six of the 114 medical schools in the United States had established department or divisions. Although ninety-three residency programs existed in hospitals affiliated with schools of medicine, only fifty-eight were in the principal university hospitals. *

The Coordinating Council on Medical Education (CCME) †
published a report in September 1975 encouraging medical schools to accept greater responsibility for providing an appropriate environment to motivate students to select careers related to the teaching and practice of primary care.[4] A primary care physician was defined as

. . . one who establishes a relationship with an individual or family for which he provides continuing surveillance of their health care needs, comprehensive care for the acute and chronic disorders which he is qualified to care for, and access to the health care delivery system for those disorders requiring the services of other specialists.[5]

The report recommended that

. . . institutions responsible for graduate education, including university hospitals, should be encouraged to establish residencies in family practice, internal medicine and pediatrics with orientation toward primary care.[6]

Among other recommendations was one that directed the American boards of internal medicine and pediatrics

. . . to re-examine their requirements for admission to their certifying

---

* Robert Graham, 24 July 1975: personal communication.
† The parent bodies of the CCME are: American Board of Medical Specialties, American Hospital Association, American Medical Association, Association of American Medical Colleges, and Council of Medical Specialty Societies.

examinations so that educational programs and careers of internists and pediatricians interested in primary care will have at least the same professional prestige as subspecialty categories of internal medicine and pediatrics.[7]

The American Board of Internal Medicine is in the process of changing its structure and requirements so that residencies will be viewed by potential candidates for board certification as an entity, and less as a preparation for fellowship in one of the subspecialities such as cardiology or hematology.

Medical students and recent graduates are displaying an easily demonstrable interest in careers in primary care. United States graduates entering first-year positions in family practice, internal medicine, and pediatrics rose from 32.2 percent in 1968[8] to 43.5 percent in 1973.[9]

Lack of qualified faculty has presented a serious problem in the development of departments of family medicine in schools of medicine. This has been overcome in part by internists, psychiatrists, and pediatricians assisting in the instruction of students. While their participation in the educational process is essential, it does not contribute to the development of the appropriate image of a family practitioner, which is highly desirable for purposes of professional identification in university medical centers.

The future of family practice is unknown. The specialty has had an excellent beginning, and it is expanding in terms of the numbers of physicians identified, and indeed certified, as family practitioners. The future will be determined by the academic stature of the specialty in university medical centers, and the professional satisfactions of daily practice.

FOREIGN MEDICAL GRADUATES (FMGs)

For the past ten years the public and the medical profession have become progressively more aware of the increasing number of foreign medical graduates coming to this country for graduate medical education. Upward of 70 percent of them remain here, in either individual or institutional practice. Within the past two to three years, however, the implications of this large ingress of FMGs has been discussed more openly by Congress and the national professional organizations.

The number of FMGs in this country increased from 36,569 in 1963 to 77,660 in 1973, an increment of 112.3 percent;[10] the growth rate for graduates of United States medical schools was 21 percent in the same period.

There were 2,072 FMGs in internship and residency positions in this country in 1950–51, whereas in 1973–74 there were 18,348,[11] an increment of almost 800 percent.

In 1963, 1,451 FMGs received licenses to practice medicine: 17.5 percent of the total number of newly licensed physicians. In 1973 the 7,419 FMGs licensed represented 44.5 percent of the total; [12] over 50 percent of new licentiates in nineteen states were FMGs.

FMGs occupy over 50 percent of the filled positions in residencies in anesthesiology, pathology, and physical medicine and rehabilitation; they hold only 7 percent of the filled positions in family practice and ophthalmology. This divergence of occupancy of residency positions probably represents a combination of the interest American graduates have in these specialties and the number of positions available.

Concern has been expressed about the quality of care delivered by FMGs. Weiss and his associates state that:

It therefore seems likely that a large number of FMGs are functioning in a medical underground delivering patient care in an unsupervised and unregulated fashion.[13]

Various estimates have been made as to the number of unlicensed FMGs—some exceed ten thousand.

The CCME, as a part of a long-range survey of physician manpower in the United States, has studied all aspects of the influx of FMGs to this country and has made a statement on the subject, embracing forty-seven recommendations addressed to medical schools, teaching hospitals, licensing bodies, certifying agencies, and several segments of the federal government.[14] The report contains general as well as specific recommendations addressed to: 1) temporary visitor-physicians; 2) foreign national physicians seeking permanent residence; 3) American nationals studying medicine abroad; and 4) United States assistance to medical education in developing countries.

In composing the report the CCME was acutely aware of the many real and alleged problems inherent in accepting thousands of FMGs each year into graduate educational programs in the United States. At no time during the development of the report was there even a suggestion of abolishing the opportunity for FMGs to participate in graduate programs in this country. On the contrary, the emphasis of the report is that:

1. Assurance be given that FMGs who want to come to this country as either exchange visitors or permanent immigrants are qualified to benefit from the type of training available;

2. The educational programs offered be under the sponsorship of schools of medicine, and therefore presumably of acceptable quality;

3. Exchange visitor-physicians be sponsored by educational institutions in their own countries;

4. Their own governments or educational institutions assure them of secure positions on their return;

5. Appropriate and effective orientation programs be required under the sponsorship of educational agencies;

6. The CCME be responsible for formulating national policies with respect to educational programs for FMGs;

7. The Liaison Committee on Graduate Medical Education (LCGME) be responsible for the accreditation of all programs, including fellowships and special programs in which FMGs are enrolled;

8. The LCGME establish for both American graduates and FMGs a single standard of competence for assuming responsibility for patient care under supervision; and

9. The CCME assume responsibility for assembling information concerning positions available for FMGs, the actual operation of the programs, and their effectiveness with respect to the goals of the FMGs.

In addition, it is recommended that the CCME be responsible for the development of improved screening procedures and comprehensive national programs designed to improve the professional and related skills of all immigrant physicians seeking to engage in the practice of medicine in the United States.

Several adjunct recommendations are made in the report concerning the need for relatively uniform eligibility requirements and qualifying procedures for all physicians seeking licenses from state medical boards, and the need for all physicians not functioning as residents or fellows in an approved graduate program to have an unrestricted license if they are engaged in the practice of medicine. Other proposals concern the need for the United States to participate more actively in world health problems by providing as much assistance as possible to developing countries in order that their systems of medical education may reach a high enough level to meet their basic health care needs.

Throughout the development of the CCME report it was recognized that a complete spectrum of professional capability existed in the FMG physician population, ranging from seventeen hundred invaluable full-time members of medical school faculties to others who will probably never be capable of passing a licensure examination. The principal purpose of the report is to establish standards of eligibility and performance that would apply in a nondiscriminatory fashion to all physicians entering graduate programs or practice. Since the report must be approved by the five parent organizations, changes may be made before the published document is available.

In April 1975 the CCME, with the Educational Commission for Foreign Medical Graduates and the National Council on International Health, sponsored a conference on "The Foreign Medical Graduate." Representatives of all voluntary health agencies concerned with FMGs participated, as did representatives from the departments of state, labor, justice, and health, education, and welfare. There was a remarkable consensus on the general principles of the report. Several pertinent suggestions for change were incorporated in the final version approved by the CCME. The CCME has strong convictions that the report address itself to every aspect of the problem; that it is fair, devoid of bias, and free of recommendations that display any vested interest; and that, if it is accepted, maximum opportunities will be provided for qualified FMGs to benefit from graduate educational programs in the United States.

THE FIRST YEAR OF GRADUATE MEDICAL EDUCATION

Early in this century the internship was the final formal educational experience of most physicians preparing for general practice. From the 1930s on, the internship changed in character as specialty residency programs became the customary educational experience after physicians had completed the internship. Rather than being the terminal educational experience, the internship became a prerequisite for admission to a residency. The 1966 Report of the Citizens Commission on Graduate Medical Education noted the existence of an undesirable discontinuity of medical education, which was manifested in the separate control and accreditation of undergraduate education, internships, and residencies.[15]

The CME presented a statement, "Continuum of Medical Education." [16] to the AMA House of Delegates in December 1970. The statement was accepted. Of ten recommendations bearing on medical education, one was designed to change certain aspects of the internship. It stated "that the first year of medical education following receipt of the M.D. degree be accredited by an appropriate residency review committee." Up until then the internship was accredited separately by the CME. Acceptance of the recommendation by the AMA permitted the integration of internships and residencies, and the elimination of internships in hospitals that did not offer residencies.

The intent was not to eliminate a year of graduate medical education, but to require the corporate consideration of the directors of clinical services in a teaching hospital to design and monitor a first year that would provide a desirable and effective experience for the graduate, depending on his career choice. This concept was most applicable to graduates desiring careers in anesthesiology, radiology, psychiatry, neurology, dermatology, and obstetrics and gynecology. In the major clinical areas such as medicine, surgery, and pediatrics, the large number of straight internships was a de facto part of the corresponding residency.

Shortly after the AMA's statement was made public, many of the specialty boards reduced the length of time required for a residency, which in effect eliminated the internship as it was then constituted. Because so many medical schools were adopting a three-year curriculum, and because of the elimination of the internship as a formal part of graduate medical education, individuals in many instances could complete their total formal undergraduate and graduate education in six years.

Program directors, especially in anesthesiology, psychiatry, and neurology, became progressively more concerned about the early differentiation of a student or graduate into a specialist without his having had a sufficiently broad exposure to the whole field of medicine. The lack of wide clinical experience and an inadequate comprehension of the patient's total problem furthered the disease or system orientation of the specialist. Sufficient dismay was expressed over this deficiency in the education of physicians that by 1975 most of the specialty boards had redefined their requirements to include a year of broad clinical experience.

This change by the specialty boards did not resolve all problems, however, since many of the new requirements for the first year included at least four months of rotation on a medical service. Directors of medical services, besieged by requests for such rotations by directors of anesthesiology, ophthalmology, dermatology, psychiatry, neurology, radiology, pathology, and obstetrics and gynecology, could not provide the required positions and still assure their own residents of adequate responsibility for patients or a meaningful educational experience. The problem has been resolved in part by departments of medicine establishing affiliations with federal and community hospitals to provide additional positions at the first-year level; departments of pediatrics have also shared the burden.

Ultimate solutions to this and many other problems related to graduate medical education in a teaching hospital will not be achieved until the directors of clinical services participate in corporate decisions made on behalf of the best interests of the institution's educational program, rather than permitting final decisions to be made on a departmental basis.

MEDICAL SCHOOLS AND GRADUATE MEDICAL EDUCATION

Formal graduate medical education became a reality in this country in the early part of the twentieth century. Internships were offered by a variety of hospitals, and, by 1910, 70 percent of the graduates were voluntarily seeking this type of post-M.D. experience. Students themselves realized that if they were to have sufficient ability and confidence to practice independently, some hospital training was needed beyond the exposure to patients obtained as undergraduates. The internships, mostly of one year's duration, were designed to prepare the physician for general practice. At the beginning of the century they were not required by either schools of medicine or state licensing bodies.

Starting with the University of Minnesota, in 1915 medical schools began to require an internship as part of the formal education of a physician; fifteen medical schools had such a requirement by 1936. This practice was discontinued, however, primarily because faculties were uncomfortable about their lack of authority over the education of interns in hospitals, many of which had no formal affiliation with a medical school and were frequently at great distances from a school. By 1955 all schools had abandoned the required internship.

When residencies in the multiple specialties began to develop in the 1920s and 1930s, informal overtures were again made to the schools of medicine to assume the responsibility for graduate as well as undergraduate education. There was essentially no response from the schools.

One of the recommendations in the 1965 Coggeshall Report stated:

> In the future, professional physician education should continue in a coordinated sequence under the sponsorship and guidance of university medical schools, through internship and residency programs.[17]

The Council of Academic Societies of the AAMC held a conference in 1968 on "The Role of the University in Graduate Medical Education." An important proposal emanating from this conference was that:

> Universities should be urged to encourage their medical faculties to assume the same sort of responsibility for graduate medical education that they have for undergraduate medical education.[18]

The AAMC itself endorsed the concept that university medical centers should ultimately assume the responsibility for graduate medical education. In 1974 it published a report, *Guidelines for Academic Medical Centers Planning to Assume Institutional Responsibility for Graduate Medical Education,* which addressed in detail such subjects as governance; administrative arrangements; selection of students; evaluation of progress; graduation; counseling; curriculum development; service and education; financing; and attitudinal development.[19]

In 1974 the CCME issued a statement requiring the assumption of corporate responsibility by institutions, organizations, or agencies that offered programs in graduate medical education.[20] It pointed out in detail the characteristics of corporate responsibility.

As might have been anticipated, the foregoing proposals were received with mixed feelings by the medical schools, affiliated and unaffiliated hospitals, specialty boards, and residency review committees. The medical schools, in general, viewed the assumption of new responsibilities in graduate education as an additional burden, in the presence of expanding undergraduate classes. Almost universally, the schools were beset with financial deficits as a result of increasing costs and inflation, and although the major cost of conducting graduate education would still be the responsibility of affiliated hospitals, the schools anticipated some increment, primarily for administration.

Although hospital administrators and governing bodies in affiliated hospitals expressed concern over the potential loss of authority in the area of graduate education, the strongest reluctance to shift the authority to schools of medicine was voiced by clinical departmental and divisional directors. For decades they had functioned as independent proprietors of their residencies, and they had rarely been questioned about their programs, even by their colleagues. There had been almost no corporate effort displayed by the directors in terms of the hospital's total educational program. Confronted with the potential of multidisciplinary faculty groups establishing goals and objectives for their residencies, as well as for curriculum design and evaluation, they expressed a considerable degree of anxiety and even adversity. Most had become comfortable with the prescriptions of their respective specialty boards, since they permitted considerable freedom and essentially no monitoring.

Unaffiliated hospitals expressed mixed feelings about a potentially compulsory relationship with a university medical center. The more successful and larger unaffiliated hospitals saw no need for a relationship, and regarded it as detracting from their existing professional stature.

Smaller unaffiliated hospitals, most of which had a limited number of approved residencies and a restricted educational capability, discerned the advantages of a university affiliation, but were apprehensive about being dominated and engulfed by the faculty and administration of a school of medicine. Practicing physicians in these hospitals were aware of the increased demands for teaching that would be required of them, and recognized that this could disrupt the efficiency and convenience of their daily professional lives, which were devoted almost exclusively to providing service to their patients. The addition of full-time faculty to the staffs of unaffiliated hospitals, essentially for educational purposes, was frequently looked upon as a competitive activity and a threat to their professional security.

The specialty boards developed in the 1920s and 1930s filled a vacuum created by medical schools that did not see fit to assume responsibility for and authority over graduate education. Over the past three decades the boards have grown in authority, not only because board certification has today attained the status of pseudo-licensure, but because the requirements of the boards for the various residency programs have shaped the entire direction and contour of graduate medical education. Some specialty boards may view the role of medical schools in graduate education as a threat to their traditional prerogatives, and this very likely will lead to some conflict in the future.

The basic purpose of specialty boards is to certify to the medical profession and to the public the competence of an individual physician about to engage in the independent practice of medicine. This certifying process will remain with the boards. They have achieved too much public and professional credibility to have any significant insecurity about the educational role of medical schools in graduate education. The certifying process not only will, but should, remain a responsibility of the boards, since criteria and standards employed in the process represent the identification of customary practices in the various specialties. The boards, although independent, in essence represent the major specialty organizations, which, through continuing attention to defining and improving the standards of patient care, provide basic support for the existence of specialty boards.

The anticipated confrontation between the boards and the medical schools on this issue has not and probably will not occur, unless and until institutional rather than existing programmatic accreditation is introduced. At present, residency review committees for each of the twenty-two major specialties review programs periodically and make recommendations for approval, probation, or disapproval to the LCGME, the accrediting agency. The "essentials" for the residencies are devised by the residency review committees, which consist in every instance of appointees from the CME, the respective specialty board, and in some instances the respective major specialty society. Each now approves the essentials, which largely represent the educational requirements of the board. There is a strong conviction among members of residency review committees, specialty boards, and specialty societies that, if medical schools are accredited as institutions to conduct graduate as well as undergraduate medical education, the quality of individual residencies will not be maintained as vigorously and as thoroughly as it now is. They are also concerned that individuals surveying a medical school may have little knowledge of or experience with the complexity of many of the specialties. Although institutional accreditation is employed in other countries without widespread expressions of dismay, it will develop slowly in this country, and only if implementation is carried out with considerable tact and exemplary thoroughness.

In spite of all the problems that either exist or are imagined, the basic logic of providing a continuum of the undergraduate and graduate parts of medical education under the authority of a chartered educational institution is too great to be permanently denied. Several schools of medicine are proceeding to plan for the administrative obligations and the faculty effort required for the assumption of responsibility for graduate education. When a few prestigious medical schools have resolved the many issues involved, the concept will gradually be accepted by others.

PHYSICIAN MANPOWER AND GRADUATE MEDICAL EDUCATION

The public's concern about the availability of comprehensive medical services, as expressed through federal and state legislative bodies, has elicited considerable attention from the medical profession over the past five years.

The present problem of physician manpower commenced in the 1950s, when the support of research by the federal government and several national professional organizations, and the progressive decimation of the major clinical specialties into subspecialties, changed the characteristics of medical school faculties and the staffs of their affiliated hospitals. The general internist and general pediatrician were eliminated from positions of favor and stature and replaced by growing numbers of cardiologists, gastroenterologists, hematologists, nephrologists, diabetologists, endocrinologists, and others whose academic advancement depended on research productivity. The image of a generalist or primary care physician in the environment of a university medical center was no longer meaningful to medical students contemplating a choice of career.

With fewer generalists being educated in medical and pediatric residencies, and the increasing attrition rate of general practitioners, the public began to realize that physicians who could and would provide continuing comprehensive care were becoming scarce. Many people, medically indigent and affluent, were having trouble finding satisfactory access to the health care system. The enormous increase in visits to emergency services throughout the country is, at least in part, a reflection of people's lack of access to a physician of their own. Between 1954 and 1973 such visits went from 9,418,755 [21] to 61,306,171,[22] a rise of 551 percent.

Initially it was thought that the problem of availability of physicians would be solved merely by increasing the number of medical school graduates. The Report of the Surgeon General of the Public

Health Service in 1959 recommended that graduates of schools of medicine and osteopathy be expanded from seventy-four hundred to eleven thousand a year.[23]

A Presidential Advisory Commission on Health Manpower recommended in 1967 that

> . . . the production of physicians should be increased beyond presently planned levels by a substantial expansion in the capacity of existing medical schools and by continued development of new schools.[24]

Between 1960 and 1973 the number of medical schools rose from eighty-six to 114, and the number of graduates from 6,994 to 11,862.[25] The increment in graduates did not, however, solve the basic problem. Proportionately more subspecialists were produced, who for the most part settled in urban areas.

Congressmen expressed the opinion that there was an insufficient number of primary care residencies and, almost as a corollary, too many surgical residencies. Aside from their concern about the large number of FMGs obtaining permanent residence status in this country, all their proposals contained mechanisms for increasing the number of physicians, especially primary care physicians.

Many national medical organizations embarked on studies to determine the anticipated need for specialists of all types. The results of many of the studies were inconclusive, since it is almost impossible to be precise in estimating the number of various specialists that may be needed in the future. Numerous factors influence a physician's choice of specialty and location of practice, many of which are not subject to manipulation.

The most extensive survey was conducted by the American Surgical Association and the American College of Surgeons. The study, *Surgery in the United States,* suggests that the approximately twenty-six hundred residents who complete their training in all surgical specialties each year are considerably in excess of what this country will require in the foreseeable future—a number between sixteen hundred and two thousand appears desirable and reasonable.[26] This recommendation takes into consideration the fact that some thirty thousand physicians who perform surgical procedures have either not been formally trained to do so or are not certified by a surgical specialty board. The report also recommends that the number of surgical residency positions be controlled.

While the study addresses the specialty distribution of surgeons in detail, it also demonstrates that the geographic distribution of surgeons, especially in general surgery, obstetrics and gynecology, orthopedics, and urology, is quite satisfactory.

Attitudes are being expressed by members of Congress that the medical profession and its educational institutions cannot solve the manpower problem because of a lack of sufficient authority vested in any single professional agency. They believe the development of policy statements by such agencies as the CCME will not be effective in changing the distribution of medical graduates by specialty. In general, the federal government favors a more centralized authority within the Department of Health, Education, and Welfare, which would determine the number of residency positions in each specialty, and use its health care reimbursement programs to enforce its policies.

This attitude on the part of federal legislators persists, even though changes that have occurred in the past two years suggest that the many segments of the medical profession are being responsive to the expressed needs of the public, especially when policies are generated and endorsed by national professional agencies.

Proportionately more medical students are seeking residencies in primary care specialties; fewer are taking surgical residencies. The number of first-year residency positions in family practice is now around sixteen hundred, and they are oversubscribed. The emphasis on general internal medicine by the American Board of Internal Medicine will change the attitudes of internists in training. It appears that marginal residency programs in all specialties are being discontinued at an accelerated rate. One major problem for all who are concerned with the adequacy of physician manpower is that the effects of policy created and implemented by the profession take several years to become visible to the people. This is true for either self-imposed professional policy or arbitrarily decreed federal regulation of residencies. Since seven years or more are required for the formal education of physicians, changes in specialty distribution must undergo a period of transition before the impact of change is appreciated in the community.

A piece of legislation passed by Congress in 1974 will probably have a significant bearing on the problem of specialty and geographic distribution of physicians. Among other innovations, the National Health Policy, Planning, and Resources Development Act of 1974 established multiple Health Service Areas within which

Health Service Agencies (HSAs) would have the responsibility for: 1) improving the health of individuals residing in the HSA's area; 2) expanding the accessibility, acceptability, continuity, and quality of health services provided them; and 3) restraining increases in the cost of providing health services.[27]

In order to achieve these objectives a detailed analysis of existing services, facilities, and health professional manpower is required. Efforts of this nature are badly needed, since the number and types of physicians can be determined effectively only on the basis of the documented adequacy or inadequacy of health care provided in a defined medical service area.

The arbitrary regulation of graduate medical education by the delineation of numbers, types, and locations of residencies, by either the federal government or voluntary medicine, is very apt to be counterproductive unless the policies devised, and their implementation, are based on a much more objective analysis of the quantity and quality of medical services presently being provided to well-defined regional areas. The only demonstrable and documented issues concerning physician manpower at the present are that the entire country needs more primary care physicians and less dependence on the annual introduction of thousands of FMGs. These two problems and their solutions are being pursued vigorously by voluntary medicine.

It would be unfortunate in a democratic society for the federal government to preempt the long-standing prerogatives of voluntary medicine, especially since its responsiveness to social need is more than evident at the present time.

Notes

1. "Medical Education in the United States," *Journal of the American Medical Association* 194 (November 1965): 772.
2. Anne E. Crowly, ed., "Medical Education in the United States, 1973–74," *Journal of the American Medical Association,* suppl. 231 (January 1975): 47.
3. *Meeting the Challenge of Family Practice,* Report of the Ad Hoc Committee on Education for Family Practice of the Council on Medical Education (Chicago: American Medical Association, 1966).
4. "Physician Manpower and Distribution. The Primary Care Physician," Report of the Coordinating Council on Medical Education, *Journal of the American Medical Association* 233 (August 1975): 880.
5. Ibid.
6. Ibid.
7. Ibid.

8. *Directory of Approved Internships and Residencies. 1969–70* (Chicago: American Medical Association, 1970).

9. *Directory of Approved Internships and Residencies. 1974–75* (Chicago: American Medical Association, 1975).

10. *Distribution of Physicians in the United States, 1973* (Chicago: American Medical Association, Center for Health Services Research and Development, 1974): 42.

11. Crowley, ed., "Medical Education, 1973–74," p. 49 (see note 2).

12. "Medical Licensure 1973. Statistical Reviews," *Journal of the American Medical Association* 229 (July 1974): 245.

13. R. J. Weiss, et al., "Foreign Medical Graduates and the Medical Underground," *New England Journal of Medicine* 290 (June 1974): 1408.

14. *Physician Manpower and Distribution. The Foreign Medical Graduate,* Report of the Coordinating Council on Medical Education (To be published).

15. J. S. Millis, *The Graduate Education of Physicians,* Report of the Citizens Commission on Graduate Medical Education (Chicago: American Medical Association, 1966).

16. "Continuum of Medical Education," *Journal of the American Medical Association* 218 (November 1971): 1251.

17. Lowell T. Coggeshall, *Planning for Medical Progress Through Education* (Evanston, Illinois: Association of American Medical Colleges, 1965).

18. C. McC. Smythe, T. D. Kinney, and M. H. Littlemeyer, "The Role of the University in Graduate Medical Education," *Journal of Medical Education* 44, spec. iss. (September 1969).

19. *Guidelines for Academic Medical Centers Planning to Assume Institutional Responsibility for Graduate Medical Education* (Washington: Association of American Medical Colleges, 1974).

20. *CCME Policy Statement on the Responsibilities of Institutions and Organizations Offering Graduate Medical Education Programs,* Minutes of the Meeting of the Coordinating Council on Medical Education (Chicago: n.p., 18 March 1974).

21. *Journal of the American Hospital Association Guide Issue* 29 (1955).

22. *Hospital Statistics, 1974.* 1973 data from *American Hospital Association Annual Survey* (Chicago: American Hospital Association): p. 34, table V.

23. *Physicians for a Growing America,* Report of the Surgeon General's Consultant Group on Medical Education (Washington: U.S. Department of Health, Education, and Welfare, Public Health Service Publication No. 709, 1959).

24. *Report of the National Advisory Commission on Health Manpower* (Washington: U.S. Government Printing Office, November 1967).

25. "Undergraduate Medical Education," *Journal of the American Medical Association* 226 (November 1973): 903.

26. *Surgery in the United States,* A Joint Study by the American College of Surgeons and the American Surgical Association (n.p.: n.p., 1975).

27. *National Health Policy, Planning, and Resources Development of 1974,* Report by the Committee on Interstate and Foreign Commerce (Washington: U.S. Government Printing Office, 1974).

Medical Education, 1985: A Forecast

WILLIAM G. ANLYAN

In 1975, as one looks at the future of medical education in 1985, there is a analogy to living in 1950 and predicting the future of aviation in 1960. Why? The major advances made in commercial aviation by 1960 were already being tested out by the military in 1950 with the jet air force tanker that was eventually converted to the Boeing 707. And yet, despite the fact that no major new technological discovery would be needed, the nation was derelict in preparing airports, runways, and aircraft control systems for the subsonic jet age. In many ways we are in the same situation with regard to looking ahead to medical education in 1985. While the trends to be expected are already in motion, appropriate planning is lagging behind woefully.

What are some of the trends already in the process of evolution?

THE INTERFACE OF COLLEGES AND UNIVERSITIES WITH THE BASIC MEDICAL SCIENCES

There will be an increase in the opportunities for college students interested in the biological and behavioral aspects of human biology. At the undergraduate level, more colleges and universities will organize human biology courses with multiple outlets other than medicine: careers in the social sciences, such as political science, history, economics, sociology, law, and theology as they relate to health care are just a few examples. Many components of current offerings at the college level can interface with the health sciences to produce hybrids with careers in the future of the health industry.

ELIMINATION OF THE UNITRACK OF QUANTITATIVE SCIENCE AS THE ONLY POINT OF ENTRY TO MEDICAL SCHOOL

Today, 95 percent of successful entrants to medical school have followed a strict and limited unitrack of quantitative science in

270

order to compete for admission. It should be possible, with the formation of a consortium of medical schools and universities, to guarantee admission to medical school to a limited number (perhaps 25 percent of the openings) of students in their second year of college. Such provisional admission would be based on past performance, intelligence, and motivation, with the understanding that these attributes will be maintained in the ensuing years. With such an early admissions process, the basic medical sciences could be taken at random at the collegiate level. The student would feel freer to take courses other than in quantitative science, such as those in the humanities. Within two to three years, on successful completion of the minimum requirements, including the basic sciences, the student would be admitted directly into the clinical science years of medical school. Anatomy, biochemistry, and physiology, for example, could be taken at random, and not necessarily in the same year, as in a large bolus of quantitative science currently absorbed in a spectrum of time between four to nine months in certain medical schools.

THE PREMEDICAL ADVISORY SYSTEM AND MEDICAL SCHOOL ADMISSIONS COMMITTEES

In order to accomplish these objectives the premedical advisory system will have to be strengthened, with more involvement by medical school faculty in the advisory system at the collegiate level. The fear on the part of the biological, physical, and social sciences at the collegiate level that potential Ph.D. candidates in their respective fields will be "raided" by the medical schools should be minimized.

Medical school admissions committees, in turn, must be willing to accept a certain percentage of early admissions. They should give up the "sure bet" of the quantitative science, unitrack product. Today the latter is much more likely to overcome the rigorous one-to-two year bolus of basic medical sciences. With these courses being taken at random in college, prior to entrance into the clinical years, this apprehension on the part of admissions committees would be eliminated.

NUMBERS OF PHYSICIANS, AND SPECIALITY AND GEOGRAPHIC MALDISTRIBUTION

It is not possible to separate the three interrelated components necessary to have a uniform, smoothly functioning medical care system in the United States. Unlike Israel and France, we cannot afford the resources to permit "open admission" to medical school. Any qualified student in Israel has a "right" to a medical education. Despite the surplus of physicians in that relatively small country, the problems of geographic and specialty maldistribution have not been eliminated. In France, 75 percent of students admitted to the first year of the continuum of medical education are eliminated before the second year by a stiff examination. Neither of these processes should be espoused by the United States.

Through stricter reviews at the national level by residency review committees, weaker programs on chronic probation should be eliminated. Total institutional capability for providing residency training, and approval of each program by residency review committees, will continue to come under the surveillance and accreditation mechanism of the Liaison Committee on Graduate Medical Education (LCGME). Thus, as changes in the mix of types of specialty residency training are needed, they can be achieved initially by the elimination of weak programs.

The geographic maldistribution of physicians is one of the most difficult to correct in a free society such as the United States. The author, as an individual, advocates two years of national service on a mandatory basis for all graduates of medical schools, before, during, or after residency training. The service would be performed in a geographic area of need. Scholarship support and enlistment in the National Health Service Corps on a voluntary basis during the continuum of medical education may prove to be viable alternatives. The Area Health Education Centers programs, as described later in this paper, may be a third mechanism to provide exposure of medical students and resident staff to the advantages of practice in areas of need.

We must place reliance on appropriate national bodies to make ongoing studies, with the assimilation of objective data on which to look ahead five to ten years at the numbers of physicians needed. The data could be updated on a yearly roll-forward basis, to provide maximum lead time for the planning of needed resources. This would avoid the 180 degree fluctuation to which the medical schools were subjected by the federal government between 1968 and 1973. In 1968 there was said to be a "critical shortage" of physicians, and major efforts were made through the Physician Augmentation Program, and subsequently through captitation, to increase enrollment in medical schools both by the expansion of existing schools and the creation of new schools; in 1973 the Department of Health, Education, and Welfare reversed itself completely, with the official pronouncement that we had a sufficient number of physicians in the pipeline and that the principal problems were specialty and geographic maldistribution.

National bodies such as the Coordinating Council on Medical Education (CCME) or a National Commission on Medical Education should provide data from which it would be possible to project future specialty manpower needs. It is important that these national bodies be in the private sector, with participation by the federal government, in order to avoid the politicization of health manpower production. There is already in existence a mass of data accumulated by such groups as the Committee on the Study of the Surgical Services of the United States on current trends in surgical manpower production. Comparable data are available for nonsurgical specialties. Self-regulation of the numbers of approved residencies for various specialties is being advocated by such groups as the LCGME and the CCME.

CATEGORICAL AND INTERDEPARTMENTAL EDUCATIONAL PROGRAMS

It is predicted that by 1985 there will be an increase in the trend initiated at Western Reserve in the mid-1950s for a coordinated organ or categorically based interdepartmental learning experience. This has been particularly successful in the neural sciences, and it is evolving rapidly in the fields of oncology and cardiovascular disease. The same trends will prevail for electives and for medical scientist (M.D.–Ph.D.) programs. The latter will continue to form the educational base for the majority of future academic manpower, especially for clinical investigators.

On a much smaller and highly selected basis, special undertakings such as M.D.–Ph.D. programs in history, M.D.–J.D. medico-legal programs, and M.D.–M.P.H programs should be continued

On an international basis, a high-quality program for multilingual medical historians with a facility to translate ancient and medieval languages is needed, lest we lose our ability to retrieve the experiences and knowledge of the past.

THE CLINICAL LABORATORY FOR MEDICAL EDUCATION

The perimeter of the clinical laboratory for medical education will continue to expand to provide elective experiences in selective community hospitals and clinics. These will be preceptorships taken under qualified adjunct faculty. Special emphasis will be placed on education in primary medical care as it fits into the primary health care system. (This subject is covered in other chapters in this book and I shall not enlarge on it.) The Area Health Education Centers programs, such as the one in North Carolina, have served to enhance this development. Other approaches have been adopted by the WAMI program and the University of Illinois program, as described elsewhere in this volume.

THE EDUCATION OF THE FUTURE "HEALTH TEAM"

At the student level, coordinated education of various members of the "health team" will continue to take place at the bedside or in the clinic setting. It is not anticipated that there will be any greater use of formal classroom or laboratory teaching among medical students and basic science pre-Ph.D. students vis-à-vis other health professional students, except for dentistry. Continuing education programs will, however, provide expanded educational opportunities for an entire team of health professionals, rather than for each one singly in isolation. For example, the continuing educational program in renal dialysis for the health team in that field at the community level will probably be carried out in a group setting.

CORPORATE RESPONSIBILITY OF INSTITUTIONS
FOR GRADUATE MEDICAL EDUCATION

As has been advocated by various national organizations, including the CCME, and in great detail by the Association of American Medical Colleges, there will continue to be a degree of corporate responsibility for graduate medical education in teaching hospitals. This development has been enhanced by two factors: 1) a greater interdependence of one discipline on another for optimum medical care, for example, the interdependence of neurology, neuroradiology, and neurosurgery. Thus it is important to have excellence across the board; an institution cannot function efficiently if one of the three units is weak in its residency training program and faculty; and 2) limited resources in the teaching hospital concomitant with the diminution in external training support for residency programs. One chief-of-service can no longer expand his particular program as an individual entrepreneur to attract external funding. More and more of the support of the resident staff is becoming an institutional responsibility, dependent on the daily charges made to patients. Such charges are also subject to audit and questioning by external groups such as Medicare and private, third-party insurance carriers.

RECERTIFICATION

By 1985 all specialties should require mandatory recertification at least every five years. Relicensure should also keep a track record of the individual physician's efforts in continuing educational programs. Recertification should be based on the individual's past performance in the perimeter of his or her activity; it should not be a complete, qualifying, specialty board examination. In other words, if a physician who is boarded in general surgery has confined his practice to breast surgery, then the continuing competence and recertification should be limited to that field.

COMMUNICATIONS SYSTEMS AND ON-LINE INFORMATION

With the increasing complexity of medical care and the biomedical information explosion, it is imperative that the medical student, the resident, and the practicing physician in 1985 have on-line, immediate access to the latest medical information available. In view of the dependence on memory, and on textbooks and papers published several months following the accumulation of data by one group or another, it will be necessary to have pooled, accumulative data on patients with certain conditions. The current experience with the myocardial infarction research unit data base, for example, which has all the characteristics of several thousand patients with acute myocardial infarctions, is a model to adopt for other major disease groups. With this computerized data base the physician in our institutions can, on a twenty-four-hour-day basis, call in from a computer terminal and match the various characteristics of the history, physical examination, and laboratory data with the cumulative experience of alternatives of therapy in the group. Thus, in the middle of the night, the physician does not have to rely on memory, an outdated textbook, or the publication of a small series that is noncumulative since submission for publication a year or more ago. Such information is also now available on-line for consultative use by physicians in selected community hospitals and clinics. The physician of the future will therefore be more adept at the process of solving problems, rather than carrying a sheer mass of data in his head.

WHO DOES WHAT TO WHOM, WHERE, AND WHEN IN HEALTH AND MEDICAL CARE?

Today there is chaos, with over two hundred different types of persons who can be broadly classed as providers of health care: they range all the way from the telephone operator receiving a call to the physician working with many other health professionals. By 1985 it is hoped that the Institute of Medicine will have completed its study to define the roles and responsibilities of nonphysicians, health professionals, and other personnel. Currently there is a significant overlap in the relative roles and responsibilities in such areas as nurse practitioners, physician's associates, and other health professionals. The institute's study will provide a better guide to modification of medical school and residency curricula. There should be a shift to nonphysician personnel of repetitive technical responsibilities currently performed by the physician.

FINANCING THE CONTINUUM OF MEDICAL EDUCATION

Continuing medical education and recertification should be a self-financing entity, and should continue to be a tax deductible item for the practicing physician in 1985.

Graduate education is more logically financed through the Part A mechanism of the health care dollar. It is suggested that we adopt the same arbitrary decision as the United Kingdom and Sweden in financing residency training through the health care delivery system.

We are faced with the dilemma of financing undergraduate medical education. At this stage it is not possible to predict whether the federal government will continue to undergird a small part (15–25 percent) of the cost of medical education, or whether the burden of high tuition will shift completely to the student. The federal government may provide scholarship and living expenses for the student in exchange for a year-for-year repayment in the National Health Service Corps or some similar national service unit. It is indeed possible that the latter course may be an unfair disadvantage for students from the lower socioeconomic levels who seek a medical education.

It is anticipated that there will be somewhat greater support for medical education from state funds as more states recognize that private institutions need to be undergirded, and that the process of medical education can be expanded at a lower cost by subsidizing the private schools. The support of state schools should continue to grow between now and 1985, at least in parallel with inflationary costs.

We should avoid the past mistakes of Japan of having markedly private and public medical education systems. Currently in that country the quality of the pool of applicants to the private schools has gone down, since the socioeconomically disadvantaged students of higher intellect cannot afford the costly tuition of a private medical education.

In conclusion, the future for medical education in the United States by 1985 would seem to be a bright one. All the trends are currently in sight. Alternatives for decisions to be made have been spelled out.

DISCUSSION

By allowing college undergraduates to take some medical school courses, there is a danger of producing an even greater number of dissatisfied students who have no chance for admission to medical school. Anlyan replied that one way of remedying this is to develop the perihealth professions and make them more attractive to students. With the present unitract system of entering medicine, many students who see the only route closed to them, become discouraged completely and fall by the wayside.

It is important that greater emphasis be placed on the humanities in medicine, and to attract those students with liberal arts and social science backgrounds. It is naive, however, to expect that there will be more humanists merely by increasing the proportion of candidates from these disciplines. There are rigidities in every field, including the humanities. Rather, the emphasis should be on expanding our understanding of what is needed for health, socioeconomic values and ecology, for example, where decisions have to be made on patterns of action to satisfy our needs without conflict with our environment.

Turning to the medical school attrition rate, participants felt that the current 1.4 percent is too low; the schools are afraid to fail students. One reason is that medical educators still have no real grasp of the noncognitive variables. And today, of course, the schools are accountable to the courts for their admissions policies. One possible solution is some form of admissions lottery, as is used in the Netherlands. For the present, however, because of religious and societal pressures, this is out of the question.

*   *   *   *

GENERAL DISCUSSION

At this point the discussion was opened for additional comments on any of the issues raised during the conference. Among the observations were:

There are two insidious forces affecting current trends in medical education: 1) lack of a national health insurance program is forcing clinical faculty members to spend more time in private practice, thus cutting down on their teaching time; and 2) the current emphasis on goal-oriented research is influencing medical education and the formation of the curriculum, thereby reducing the authority of departmental chairmen.

Financing graduate medical education from the health care dollar may not be the best solution, because this is, in effect, an attempt to force the government to pay for the continuing education of a privileged group. It may be better to have graduate medical education totally integrated into the university, with interns and residents registered as students, paying tuition, and meeting university standards, as well as those of professional bodies.

Too little attention is being paid at the present time to the "domino effect" in medicine; the husband who is unhappy at work, for example, will abuse his wife, who in turn will mistreat their children. The entire academic medical center—physicians, nurses, social workers, and psychologists—should be involved in the treatment of such problems in "centers for family wellness." Treatment should begin with genetic and social counseling.

It is easy to repeat the cliche, "Why don't the medical schools reorder their priorities?" The fact is that the hard money base that would make changes possible has decreased sharply. The solution appears to lie in special grants for family practice programs, and the development of centers for family "wellness." Such support would help prime the pump until the rest of the health care system gears up to assume the responsibility and the costs.

Some discussants pointed out that the proposed centers for family wellness resemble some aspects of the British health care system. Such efforts have thus far stayed on the periphery. What indications are there that conditions and attitudes have changed?

The basis of this issue has been the isolation of family practice and primary care. The problems are now so overwhelming, with family practice programs being "gobbled up" by other departments that state they are interested in primary care, that there may be no time to prime the pump. The question is: If pump-priming is not the proper strategy, what is?

The discussion moved to a consideration of the obstacles that lie in the way of meeting the perceived health care needs of the population. One of the real difficulties is the fragmentation of responsibilities; segments of the health professions deal only with their own areas and needs. This fragmentation, for example, prevents the hospital from acting in a corporate way on behalf of the whole community. As the system stands now, action is taken only under the threat of imposed governmental strictures.

An even more fundamental issue is that the medical profession is disease- rather than health-oriented, and disease is a fragmentary process. Since very little of the medical school curriculum is devoted to health, it is a misnomer to term the institutions "health centers."

A move toward a concern with health can be discerned in the burgeoning interest in family practice. Other primary care specialists —pediatricians and internists—ought to follow this trend.

Participants

Joel J. Alpert, M.D.
Professor and Chairman
Department of Pediatrics
School of Medicine
Boston University
Boston City Hospital
Boston, Massachusetts

William G. Anlyan, M.D.
Vice President for Health Affairs
Duke University Medical Center
Durham, North Carolina

Joseph Ceithaml, Ph.D.
Dean of Students, Biological Sciences
The Division of the Biological
    Sciences and the Pritzker School
    of Medicine
University of Chicago
Chicago, Illinois

Robert A. Chase, M.D.
President and Director
The National Board of Medical
    Examiners
Philadelphia, Pennsylvania

D. Harold Copp, M.D., Ph.D.
Professor and Chairman
Department of Physiology
Faculty of Medicine
University of British Columbia
Vancouver, B.C., Canada

R. F. Patrick Cronin, M.D.
Dean
Faculty of Medicine
McGill University
Montreal, Quebec, Canada

Eugene S. Farley, Jr., M.D.
Professor and Director
Family Medicine Program
School of Medicine and Dentistry
University of Rochester
Rochester, New York

William J. Grove, M.D.
Executive Dean
College of Medicine
University of Illinois
Chicago, Illinois

John C. Herweg, M.D.
Associate Dean, Student Affairs
School of Medicine
Washington University
St. Louis, Missouri

William D. Holden, M.D.
*Oliver H. Payne Professor of Surgery
    and Director of the Department*
School of Medicine
Case Western Reserve University
University Hospitals
Cleveland, Ohio

Mary Jane Jesse, M.D.
*Berenson Professor of
    Pediatric Cardiology*
School of Medicine
University of Miami
Miami, Florida

Davis G. Johnson, Ph.D.
Director
Division of Student Studies
Association of American Medical
    Colleges
Washington, D.C.

281

Donald W. King, M.D.
Delafield Professor of Pathology
College of Physicians and Surgeons
Columbia University
New York, New York

Charles Odegaard, Ph.D.
*Professor of Higher Education
    and President Emeritus*
University of Washington
Seattle, Washington

Vivian Winona Pinn, M.D.
Assistant Dean for Student Affairs
School of Medicine
Tufts University
Boston, Massachusetts

Theodore T. Puck, Ph.D.
Director
Eleanor Roosevelt Institute for
    Cancer Research
*Professor of Biophysics
    and Genetics*
University of Colorado Medical
    Center
Denver, Colorado

Clayton Rich, M.D.
*Vice President for Medical Affairs
    and Dean*
School of Medicine
Stanford University
Stanford, California

Thomas B. Roos, Ph.D.
Professor of Biology
Dartmouth College
Hanover, New Hampshire

M. Roy Schwartz, M.D.
*Associate Dean for Academic Affairs
    and Director, WAMI Program*
School of Medicine
University of Washington
Seattle, Washington

Robert D. Sparks, M.D.
Chancellor
University of Nebraska Medical
    Center
Omaha, Nebraska

Louis W. Sullivan, M.D.
Dean and Director
Medical Education Program
Morehouse College
Atlanta, Georgia

Gregory L. Trzebiatowski, Ph.D.
*Assistant Dean for Medical and
    Graduate Education*
College of Medicine
The Ohio State University
Columbus, Ohio

Lawrence L. Weed, M.D.
Professor of Medicine
College of Medicine
University of Vermont
Burlington, Vermont

Representing the
Josiah Macy, Jr. Foundation

John Z. Bowers, M.D.
President

Mary E. Cunnane
Coordinator of Fellowship Programs

Elizabeth F. Purcell
Conference Coordinator and Editor

INDEX